Beat Your Irritable Bowel Syndrome In Seven Simple Steps

Paul Jenner

This book is dedicated to everyone who suffers from an irritable bowel and especially to those who shared their stories with me.

Paul Jenner trained as a journalist with the Westminster Press group, later becoming a freelance writer. He is the author of more than 30 books specializing in health issues, personal development and life skills, and has reported from all over the world. He sees IBS not as a single condition but as a group of quite different conditions, all of which can nevertheless be treated by his Seven Step Programme. His other titles include *Beat Your Pain And Find Lasting Relief, Help Yourself To Live Longer, How To Be Happier, Beat Your Depression, Be More Confident, Transform Your Life With NLP* and *Have Great Sex*. His books have been translated into several languages including French, Spanish, Dutch, German and Chinese. He has written for national newspapers including *The Daily Telegraph* and *The Observer*. When not working he enjoys hiking, mountain biking, snowboarding, swimming, sailing and windsurfing. He and his partner divide their time between England, Spain and France. He would be delighted to hear from you on his website www.pauljenner.eu.

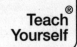
Teach Yourself®

Beat Your Irritable Bowel Syndrome In Seven Simple Steps

Paul Jenner

First published in Great Britain in 2014 by Hodder & Stoughton. An Hachette UK company.

First published in US in 2014 by The McGraw-Hill Companies, Inc.

This edition published 2014

British Library Cataloguing in Publication Data: a catalogue record for this title is available from the British Library.

Library of Congress Catalog Card Number: on file.

10 9 8 7 6 5 4 3 2 1

Cover image © Yeko Photo Studio / Shutterstock

Typeset by Cenveo® Publisher Services.

Printed and bound in Great Britain by CPI Group (UK) Ltd., Croydon, CR0 4YY.

Hodder & Stoughton policy is to use papers that are natural, renewable and recyclable products and made from wood grown in sustainable forests. The logging and manufacturing processes are expected to conform to the environmental regulations of the country of origin.

Hodder & Stoughton Ltd

338 Euston Road

London NW1 3BH

www.hodder.co.uk

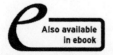

Acknowledgements

A very special thank you to Victoria Roddam and Sam Richardson, my editors at Hodder.

Contents

Introduction

IBS is not a term I like. I use it because it's well-recognized and it's short. I don't like it because when a doctor utters those three letters it makes it sound as if you've received a specific diagnosis. That's not the case at all.

IBS stands for irritable bowel syndrome, a horrible, painful, demoralizing *group* of conditions that are vaguely linked by having the same or similar symptoms. In fact, that's precisely what a syndrome is. It's a group of symptoms, not a disease. Being told you have IBS says nothing about the cause of your problems and does little to bring a successful treatment any nearer.

By comparison with your heart your digestive tract is vastly complicated. A heart is just a pump and people have been making pumps for a couple of thousand years or more. No one ever has made, or ever will make, a digestive tract. It doesn't only process food. It's also the biggest immune system organ in your body, probably responsible for something like 80 per cent of your defences. That's because it's part of the *outside* of your body, just as much as the skin of your arms. Every time you swallow you despatch all kinds of pathogens to attack it. No wonder the treatment of IBS can be so difficult.

Some doctors, the most rigorous, may insist the term IBS applies only to the failure of the muscles of the large intestine to contract and relax in a properly coordinated manner causing bloating, pain, sometimes enormous pain, and either diarrhoea or constipation or both. Others might consider, say, a dozen different conditions under the IBS umbrella. Sometimes a condition that was considered to be 'IBS' is made into a new disease. That happened with small intestinal bacterial overgrowth (SIBO). At one time hailed as *the* cause of IBS in the majority of instances, it was later 'downgraded' to be just *a* cause among numerous others, and now many doctors and gastroenterologists consider it to be a completely separate condition altogether. So there's nothing very precise about IBS. That's why I prefer to talk simply of an 'irritable bowel' (although angry bowel, furious bowel or demented bowel might be more appropriate). It's a suitably vague term for a vague group of disorders.

In practice, more than 20 separate conditions are frequently 'diagnosed' as IBS. And yet each is quite distinct. None of those conditions is life-threatening but they're all life-destroying precisely because they play havoc with probably the most fundamental part of your body.

In this book my aim is to focus on that score or so of conditions and to refine their treatment down to seven simple steps. I call it the Seven Step Programme. No matter which specific condition or combination of conditions you're suffering from those seven steps will solve your problems.

Some of the treatments will straight away, no doubt, strike you as perfectly logical. You'll enthusiastically give them a go. Others might seem illogical, bizarre or perverse. But there is science and experience behind all of them. So don't leave anything out. Begin at Step 1 and work your way methodically through the succeeding steps until you are better.

I wish you good luck with the Seven Step Programme.

Paul Jenner

England 2014

1

Step 1: Understand your IBS

In this chapter you will learn:

- ▶ *what causes an irritable bowel*
- ▶ *how your digestive system works and why it sometimes goes wrong*
- ▶ *the Seven Steps to a successful treatment.*

There's a solution to your irritable bowel problems. And it might come as soon as today. But even if there are setbacks and disappointments and false trails followed and abandoned, in the end it will be beaten. With persistence you and this book together will find a solution.

Never doubt it.

If you've already been to a doctor, or possibly several doctors, you may have been told you have IBS (irritable bowel syndrome) and that there's no cure for it. You may have read the same in books or on the internet. Well, that's simply not true. How can I say that so confidently? I say it because IBS is not a disease. A syndrome is a collection of symptoms. That's all.

Being told you have IBS is only half way between a description and a diagnosis. It's as if you went to the doctor complaining of a recurring pain above your right eye and were told you had a headache.

Recurring headaches can have several causes and it's the same with an irritable bowel. Some of the causes of an irritable bowel are definitely curable and all of them are treatable. When we know more, the term 'IBS' will probably disappear. In its place will be several defined conditions, some of which already have cures, while the rest will have cures one day.

The medical profession is in a state of flux over IBS. There are those who say IBS is quite specifically a loss of co-ordination in the muscles of the gut (which is why IBS is sometimes referred to as 'spastic colon' or 'irritable colon'). Others use IBS as an umbrella term to cover what's left when other identifiable diseases have been eliminated. As a sufferer it doesn't really matter to you what terminology is used. You're suffering discomfort, you're in pain, you're embarrassed, you're worried, your life is being spoilt and you want the symptoms to go away, whatever the cause or causes (because several problems can sometimes act together). You want to be cured. And you can be.

Have I got IBS?

Many irritable bowel sufferers tell me they were relieved when they got a 'diagnosis' of IBS because at least they knew 'what was wrong'. But, in reality, hearing that you have IBS is a long way from knowing what's wrong. The problem with the phrase 'irritable bowel syndrome' is that it makes something vague sound like something quite specific. IBS is not specific. Nevertheless it's the term you'll hear again and again when dealing with the medical profession. So let's see how IBS is assessed.

Probably your doctor will use the Rome III criteria. These have nothing to do with Rome as a place but with the so-called Rome Foundation, a non-profit organization whose stated mission is specifically to improve the lives of people with functional gastrointestinal disorders (FGIDs), of which IBS is said to be one. A 'diagnosis' of IBS under Rome III requires:

▶ Recurrent abdominal pain or discomfort at least three days a month for at least the last three months

Plus two of the following:

▶ Improvement in symptoms following defecation

▶ Change in the frequency of defecation

▶ Change in the appearance of the stools.

I prefer simply to talk of an irritable bowel because it's a vague term for a vague condition (or rather, a large number of specific conditions that are all lumped together). However, when I'm discussing the work of researchers or other members of the medical profession I'll use 'IBS' because that's the term they use. To see if you have an irritable bowel answer the following ten questions.

Diagnostic test

1 Do you experience bloating?

2 Do you have abdominal pain?

3 Is the pain worse after eating?

4 Is the urge to defecate sometimes embarrassingly urgent?

5 Is the pain relieved for a while after a bowel movement?

6 Do you feel as if evacuation of the bowel was incomplete?

7 Is there any blood or mucous in your stools?

8 Do you suffer from constipation or diarrhoea or both alternately? (Check with the Bristol Stool Scale Chart in Figure 1.1 below.)

9 Do you feel nauseous before or after bowel movements?

10 Do you suffer from any of the following: frequent headaches, fatigue, backache and muscular pains, poor appetite, quickly feeling full, belching, heartburn, frequent urination?

Bristol Stool Chart

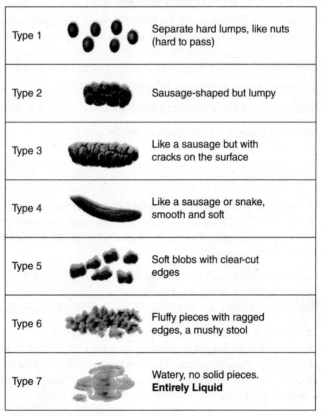

Type 1		Separate hard lumps, like nuts (hard to pass)
Type 2		Sausage-shaped but lumpy
Type 3		Like a sausage but with cracks on the surface
Type 4		Like a sausage or snake, smooth and soft
Type 5		Soft blobs with clear-cut edges
Type 6		Fluffy pieces with ragged edges, a mushy stool
Type 7		Watery, no solid pieces. **Entirely Liquid**

Figure 1.1 The Bristol Stool Scale Chart

What's included in this book?

The idea of this book is to be as comprehensive as possible. You have irritable bowel symptoms and you want them treated. It doesn't matter if they have other names or what causes them. You want them sorted and, if possible, you want them cured.

If your irritable bowel is caused by any of the following or comes into any of the following categories this book is for you:

➤ **Intestinal spasms.** The muscles of the small and large intestines don't work in a smooth and coordinated manner. Food being digested doesn't churn and advance as it should. The result is discomfort and pain.

➤ **Dysbiosis.** Too many 'bad' bacteria and not enough 'good' bacteria. Symptoms include bloating, gas and pain. Treatment is via probiotics (food and supplements containing 'good' bacteria) and diet.

➤ **Faulty transporters.** A problem with the transporters that carry nutrients across the epithelium (gut lining) may mean that certain foods can't be tolerated. Treatment is through diet.

➤ **Small intestinal bacterial overgrowth (SIBO).** SIBO means you have bacteria growing in a part of the gut that should be virtually sterile. The symptoms include gas and abdominal pain. Treatment is by diet alone, or together with a special antibiotic.

➤ **Enzyme deficiency.** Enzymes are catalysts. That's to say they speed up chemical reactions. Without the right enzymes your food will never be digested. Symptoms of deficiency include abdominal pain, bloating, gas and incompletely digested food in the stools.

▶ **Lactose intolerance**. An inability to digest lactose, a type of sugar mainly found in milk and dairy products. Symptoms include abdominal bloating, wind and diarrhoea. Lactose intolerance can be identified by a breath or blood test. Treatment is the avoidance of food or drink containing lactose.

▶ **Gluten intolerance**. Gluten is what's known as a 'protein composite' and is found in wheat, barley, rye and certain other members of the grass family. Intolerance produces the classic irritable bowel symptoms of bloating, diarrhoea and abdominal discomfort or pain. Extreme sensitivity is known as coeliac disease.

▶ **Food allergy or intolerance**. For a variety of reasons you may not be able to cope with some of the foods that other people eat without problems. Lactose and gluten are just two kinds of intolerance but there are many others. Symptoms may include bloating, gas, abdominal pain, diarrhoea, skin rashes, breathing difficulties and headaches. Treatment includes, first of all, cutting out problem foods then trying to correct the cause of the abnormal reaction (see 'leaky gut' below).

▶ **Weak stomach acid**. It means that harmful bacteria aren't killed and that protein is improperly digested. Symptoms may include abdominal pain, bloating, incompletely digested food in the stool, frequent stomach upsets and allergies. Treatment is acid supplementation.

▶ **Leaky gut**. The wall of your gut has to be permeable to nutrients, otherwise you'd die of starvation, but impermeable to toxins and dangerous bacteria, otherwise you'd die for different reasons. That's not always an easy balancing act and sometimes it goes wrong. If your gut wall sometimes allows undigested food and other undesirable particles to leak through then your immune system goes into overdrive attacking not only the dangerous particles but also, on occasion, your own body. Treatment is to restore the health of the gut through diet.

- **Gastroesophageal reflux disease (GERD).** A condition in which some of the stomach contents leak backwards into the oesophagus, causing heartburn and nausea and, sometimes, difficulty swallowing. It should help if you avoid problem foods and NSAID painkillers such as ibuprofen. Your doctor will probably prescribe acid-suppressing proton pump inhibitors or H2 blockers but, in fact, the underlying cause of GERD is usually a lack of stomach acid requiring supplementation.

- **Excess mast cells.** If you suffer from hay fever, allergic skin rashes, or have dramatic reactions to bee stings you probably already know about mast cells. As part of the immune response, mast cells release histamine and other inflammatory chemicals in a process known as degranulation causing, for example, hay fever or skin rashes. But mast cells are also distributed throughout the digestive tract. Researchers (Barbara G *et al* as well as O'Sullivan M *et al*) have found that irritable bowel sufferers have abnormally large numbers of mast cells in their digestive tracts, especially in the first part of the large intestine. This means that if you're allergic to certain foods you may have a powerful reaction actually within your intestines leading to alterations in sensitivity and gut physiology. Stress also activates these mast cells.

- **Inflammation.** It was always believed IBS patients had no inflammation in their digestive tracts. That's now been shown to be untrue. The inflammation is microscopic (which is why it was missed for years) but significant. Inflammation in the digestive tract can be treated by diet.

- **Intestinal parasites.** They can cause tenderness of the stomach, abdominal pain, diarrhoea, nausea, vomiting and bloating. Once identified by a test, the majority are easily eradicated by the appropriate medicament prescribed by your doctor.

- **Sorbitol overuse.** Sorbitol and other artificial sweeteners, laxatives or antacids can cause a variety of problems including abdominal pain, diarrhoea and weight loss. Treatment is to cut back.

- ▶ **Bile acid diarrhoea (BAD).** This is the result of overproduction of bile acid which passes into the large intestine and causes frequent watery stools. It can be treated with cholestyramine.

- ▶ **Straining to go to the toilet.** Straining leads not only to haemorrhoids but also to a variety of intestinal problems including SIBO (see above). Treatments include diet, exercise and the use of the squatting position to defecate.

- ▶ **Lack of exercise.** Humans were designed to move. When you take vigorous exercise your digestive tract gets a beneficial massage. If you don't get much exercise now then beginning an exercise programme could make a significant difference to your irritable bowel symptoms.

- ▶ **Endometriosis.** This is a condition in which the kind of material that lines the womb grows on other organs such as the ovaries or fallopian tubes. If the material grows on the intestines it can cause inflammation and pain, especially at the time of menstruation. Treatment may involve painkillers, hormones and surgery to remove the material.

- ▶ **Hormones.** If you're a woman you've probably noticed that your irritable bowel symptoms are worse around the time of your period. You may also have noticed a connection with starting the contraceptive pill, or stopping it, or switching brands. But men can have hormone-related irritable bowel symptoms, too. Treatment is to get the hormone situation right.

- ▶ **Yeast.** If *Candida albicans* grows out of control in the digestive system it can cause the classic irritable bowel symptoms as well as thrush and other problems. Treatment is an antifungal.

- ▶ **Weakness of the migrating motor complex (MMC).** The MMC sweeps everything out of the small intestine. If it's weak, bacteria can flourish, leading to SIBO (see above). Treatment may involve a prokinetic drug that stimulates movement.

- ▶ **Serotonin.** Too much of this hormone in the gut causes diarrhoea while too little causes constipation. Treatment is a serotonin modulating drug.

- .**Trauma and stress**. Extreme cases of anxiety and fear, especially over a long period or at an early age, can lead to an increase in the sensitivity of the nerves in the gut or to an increased response in the brain. Treatment may include counselling, biofeedback, hypnotherapy, self-hypnosis, Cognitive Therapy (CT) and Neuro-Linguistic Programming (NLP).

- **Irritable bowel symptoms for reasons unknown**. Even if the cause of your irritable bowel symptoms can't be pinned down there are treatments in this book that should reduce or eliminate your problems.

How your digestive system works – and sometimes goes wrong

A huge amount goes on in the digestive tract and in a way it's not at all surprising if bloating, gas, discomfort and pain are the results. What's more amazing is that we're usually so little aware of the litres of digestive juices that are squirted into our digestive tracts and of the thousands of muscular contractions and relaxations that every day turn the macerated food over and over and propel it through tubes that, spread out, would go across the width of a tennis court. So let's take a look at what happens inside your abdomen and how those irritable bowel symptoms can result (see Figure 1.2).

THE MOUTH

The mouth and its associated parts (tongue, teeth, salivary glands) form the first part of your digestive system. Use it properly. In 24 hours you produce an astonishing 1 to 1.5 litres of saliva and it's there for various reasons, in particular to begin the process of breaking down starch. If things don't go right at the beginning of the digestive process they're likely to get worse further down the line. So spend time on this stage and eat calmly to avoid swallowing air. Most swallowed air is released by burping but if even a little is retained it can only make bloating worse.

THE OESOPHAGUS

The oesophagus, the tube leading to the stomach, is the next part of the digestive system. It's not directly involved in irritable bowel

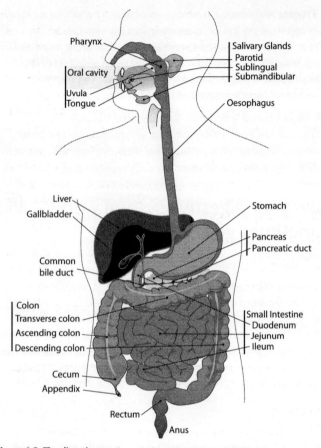

Figure 1.2 The digestive tract

symptoms, but sufferers often also have heartburn or the more relentless gastroesophageal reflux disease (GERD), caused by the failure of the lower oesophageal sphincter to close properly. That failure allows stomach acid to splash up into the oesophagus, where it shouldn't be, and cause a burning sensation. If you take some kind of antacid to tackle the symptoms (the burning sensation) you're not correcting the underlying problem (which is the failure of the valve to close). What's worse, the antacids reduce the acidity of the stomach, and that, as we'll see, could indirectly contribute to an irritable bowel.

THE STOMACH

When food arrives in the stomach it initially remains in the top part, known as the fundus. Presently, what are known as mixing waves pass over the stomach every 15 to 25 seconds, macerating the food and turning it into a thin liquid called chyme. As digestion proceeds these waves become more and more powerful, forcing a few millilitres of chyme at a time into the duodenum, the first part of the small intestine.

The stomach is an acid environment, with a pH of between one and five, depending on whether it's empty or full and what food has been eaten. Seven is neutral. Anything below seven is acid and anything above seven is alkaline (also known as basic). The acidity plays a role in several functions, including:

▶ the digestion of protein

▶ the destruction of microbes in food

▶ closing the lower oesophageal sphincter

▶ relaxing the pyloric sphincter, between the stomach and the small intestine.

When stomach acid is weak (a condition known as hypochlorhydria or, if it's non-existent, achlorhydria) five very important things can go wrong:

▶ Problem 1

The autonomic nervous system doesn't close the lower oesophageal sphincter properly because it works in response to rising acid. It's weak stomach acid that leads to a leaky valve, which is why antacids are generally (but not always) the wrong approach. The real solution is to make the stomach more acid, not less. A study published in the Journal of the American Medical Association found that medicaments to suppress stomach acid were also associated with increased risk of hip fractures, pneumonia, and age-related macular degeneration.

▶ Problem 2

The pyloric sphincter, the valve at the bottom of the stomach that holds back food until it has been sufficiently digested, only *opens* when the acid level is high enough. So low stomach acid can mean that food is retained longer in the stomach, thus causing bloating. The worst culprit is meat, especially fatty meat, which can remain in the stomach for four to six hours. (At the other extreme, water and alcohol pass through an empty stomach into the small intestine in seconds.) In certain individuals, fat in the stomach (and in the small intestine – see below) causes relatively violent movements of the large intestine (to make space for the incoming meal), causing pain. So a low-fat diet could be one solution to that irritable bowel symptom.

▶ Problem 3

Certain minerals and vitamins, especially vitamin B12, don't digest properly in weak acid, causing malnutrition.

▶ Problem 4

When stomach acid is too weak it's insufficient to kill bacteria in food, thus allowing the microbes to pass into the small intestine where they may cause illness and, for reasons we'll see in a minute, even more bloating.

▶ Problem 5

Protein is broken down into amino acids in the stomach and in the upper part of the small intestine. The amino acids pass through the wall of the gut into the bloodstream which distributes them around the body. When the hydrochloric acid in the stomach is weak not all the protein gets broken down as it should, allowing whole proteins into the bloodstream. The body wants amino acids, not whole proteins, and these are identified as enemies, leading to allergic reactions such as headaches, skin rashes and swellings, nausea, breathing difficulties and, in extreme cases, even death. They may also include the classic irritable bowel symptoms of abdominal swelling and pain with wind and diarrhoea.

So that's how irritable bowel symptoms, and other problems, may be caused by weak stomach acid. And in many cases there's a very simple solution. All you need to do is take the acid supplement Betaine HCL, or, alternatively, apple cider vinegar (ACV). Refer to Step 2 for full details.

THE SMALL INTESTINE

So what you've eaten now finds its way, semi-digested, into your small intestine together with whatever you've drunk (say two litres), the litre or more of saliva and the two litres of gastric juice, where it's all joined by a litre of bile, two litres of pancreatic juice and a litre of intestinal juice. That makes a total of nine litres. Of course, it's spread over 24 hours, but even so it's enough to bloat anybody to gigantic proportions. The reason it doesn't is that most of it, about eight litres, is absorbed into the blood capillaries once it's done its job. But some kind of malfunction in that absorption process could be another cause of bloating.

The small intestine is about 2.5 cm in diameter and 6.5 m long and chyme passes through in little packets which are churned around in a muscular process known as segmentation and propelled forward by a different muscular action known as peristalsis. A failure of coordination here can cause pain.

As to gas, that's largely produced by the action of bacteria. Here's the next important point. You shouldn't have many bacteria in your small intestine. We've already seen one way they can get in, that is, if you have weak stomach acid. The other way is from the opposite end. The bacteria work their way up from the large intestine, where they're needed, to the small intestine, where they're not. The result is what's known as small intestinal bacterial overgrowth (SIBO) and we'll be looking at diets for correcting it in Step 4.

THE LARGE INTESTINE

Having gone through the small intestine, most of what you've eaten has now been digested. But there's an important exception and it's another key to the IBS story and its treatment through diet. The exception is fibre which is not much digested in the small intestine. That fibre is fermented, that's to say, broken down, by bacteria that live in the large intestine, and that process creates large amounts of gas. So the solution to gas would seem to be to avoid high fibre foods. We'll also be examining that proposition in Step 4.

Key idea

Your gut is, in a sense, outside your body. It's the biggest part of your immune system and it's constantly under attack from the microorganisms you swallow along with your food. It has to defend you and sometimes those defences go wrong.

Remember this

IBS is a 'diagnosis' of exclusion. That's to say, it tells you what you haven't got but not very much about what you have got. If your doctor says you have IBS that means you haven't got coeliac disease, diverticulitis, gallbladder problems, bowel cancer or inflammatory bowel disease (IBD), of which the two main types are ulcerative colitis and Crohn's disease. Some doctors also use the term IBS to exclude certain other conditions such as SIBO and BAD, while others might include them under the IBS umbrella. So IBS is a vague term masquerading as something specific, which is why this book prefers to talk simply of an 'irritable bowel'.

10 questions and answers about irritable bowels

▶ Question 1: Is there a test for IBS?

Remember that IBS is not a disease but simply a collection of symptoms, so there's no test for it. However, researchers at the Sahlgrenska Academy at the University of Gothenburg, Sweden, concluded that IBS sufferers have high levels of secretogranin II and low levels of chromogranin B in their stools. Granins are a family of proteins. If this finding is confirmed then it would not only allow the accurate diagnosis of IBS but also revolutionize the whole approach. However, it seems unlikely that would apply to more than a small proportion of irritable bowel cases.

▶ Question 2: Is there just one type of IBS?

IBS is generally categorized as:

▶ IBS-D: diarrhoea predominates

▶ IBS-C: constipation predominates

- IBS-M or IBS-A: a mixture of diarrhoea and constipation (they alternate)

- Pi-IBS: post-infectious IBS, meaning that it seems to be triggered by some kind of gut infection. Pi-IBS can be IBS-D, IBS-C or IBS-M/A.

- IBS-U: unsubtyped, meaning it could be any of the above.

▶ Question 3: How can I have diarrhoea and constipation at the same time?

You have hard, impacted stools blocking the rectum, which means that nothing solid can pass and you're constipated. However, liquid can find its way around the blockage, producing attacks of diarrhoea.

▶ Question 4: Are irritable bowel symptoms the same for everyone?

The severity of symptoms varies enormously. Some people have just a few attacks a year while others wrestle with the problem every single day. Some people suffer only mild pain while others go through agony that has been likened to childbirth. Some people have diarrhoea three or four times a day while others can't ever be further than a minute from a toilet and still others go only once a week.

▶ Question 5: How common is IBS?

Based on visits to doctors, it's estimated that 10 per cent of the UK population and 14 per cent of the USA population is affected. But given that many people are too embarrassed to seek medical assistance the true figures could be much higher. Some experts put it around 20 per cent.

▶ Question 6: Why me?

It's estimated that 20 to 30 per cent of all cases of IBS follow an infection that caused diarrhoea, especially acute infectious gastroenteritis. This is known as post-infectious IBS (Pi-IBS).

Gastroenteritis is inflammation of the stomach and small intestine. Infectious gastroenteritis may be caused by viruses (rotavirus, norovirus, adenovirus or astrovirus), bacteria (most commonly *Escherichia coli, Salmonella, Shigella* and *Campbylobacter* species), or parasitic protozoans (notably *Giardia lamblia*).

The mechanism isn't clear but in various studies between 7 and 33 per cent of normal people do go on to develop IBS in the aftermath of acute infectious gastroenteritis. The longer the diarrhoea continues, and the more stress the person is under, the more likely Pi-IBS is.

One theory is that the infection causes an overgrowth of 'bad' bacteria in the gut. Another is that infection causes an increase in the sensitivity of the nerves of the gut which somehow becomes permanent.

It's also possible that an irritable bowel is not so much caused by the infection as by the antibiotics used to treat the infection. A study of 580,000 children over an eight-year period found that those who had been prescribed at least one course of antibiotics before the age of four were twice as likely to develop IBS as children who hadn't had antibiotics. They were also three and a half times more at risk of Crohn's disease. The risk of gut disorders rose 12 per cent with every course prescribed. A possible explanation would be that antibiotics alter gut flora, destroying 'good' bacteria and allowing 'bad' bacteria to proliferate.

Acute infectious gastroenteritis is not the only thing that can trigger irritable bowel symptoms. A significant proportion of IBS sufferers date the onset of IBS to an emotional trauma such as a death in the family or divorce (see the entry on stress, below).

A clue that IBS might have a genetic component came from a study by the Mayo Clinic in 2003. Doctors at the clinic noted that sufferers were often in the same family. But was it environmental or genetic? By looking at the medical histories of those who were blood relatives and those who were related only through marriage the researchers found that IBS occurred in 17 per cent of the patients' relatives compared with 7 per cent of the spouses' relatives. In other words, blood relatives of an IBS sufferer are themselves more than twice as likely to have irritable bowel symptoms as the relatives of the sufferer's partner. But although that suggests a genetic link environmental factors could still explain it. As at the date of writing no one has yet discovered an IBS gene but there are a number of potential candidates, notably TNFSF15 and HLA-DQ2/8.

Remember this

If you have gallstones you have a high possibility of suffering irritable bowel symptoms. But if you have your gallbladder removed you still have a high possibility of irritable bowel symptoms and an especially strong likelihood of diarrhoea. Over half a million Americans have their gallbladders removed every year and, for many of them, it's completely unnecessary. If you've been told your irritable bowel symptoms are due to gallstones do not agree to surgery without trying diet first. Gallbladder problems are beyond the scope of this book but, in general, the idea is to cut down on fried foods and fat (especially saturated fats and trans fats), dairy and gluten (principally in wheat, barley and rye). It helps to use flax oil and drink beet and cucumber juice.

Key idea

When it comes to working out why anything happens, human beings have a major design fault. They love to find 'the solution' to any problem. It has to be just *one* thing. And that sometimes blinds them to the real answer. The idea that a problem could arise from a combination of causes is very unsatisfactory to most people. But, nevertheless, it's entirely possible that your irritable bowel could be due to several factors acting together.

▶ Question 7: What is meant by IBS being a 'functional disorder'?

The medical profession has always called IBS a 'functional disorder' meaning that there's no difference between the digestive organs of 'normal' people and IBS sufferers. It was believed that, for some other reason, the digestive system just didn't *function* the way it should. We now know the digestive organs of sufferers differ in at least two ways from those of non-sufferers. One is the increased number of mast cells, notably in the first part of the large intestine. The other is microscopic inflammation.

Mast cells are involved in smooth muscle function, which means they could have something to do with the increased sensitivity of irritable bowel sufferers. They're also involved in allergic reactions. The more mast cells the more powerful those reactions are likely to be.

Inflammation is a characteristic of inflammatory bowel disease (IBD), of which the two main types are Crohn's disease and ulcerative colitis, but until recently it was not thought to play a role in IBS. The symptoms of both types of IBD include abdominal pain, internal cramps and spasms, diarrhoea, vomiting, rectal bleeding, weight loss and anaemia.

Then in 2002, researchers at the Wakefield Hospital, Wellington, New Zealand (Chadwick VC *et al*) examined colonoscopic biopsies from 77 IBS patients and compared them with 28 samples from people who had no irritable bowel symptoms. They found that 31 of the IBS patients had nonspecific microscopic inflammation, seven had lymphocytic colitis, that's to say an accumulation of white blood cells in the lining of the colon, and the remainder all had some abnormalities as compared with the control group.

It's significant that when patients with IBD are in remission, they exhibit symptoms very much the same as in IBS. In some cases IBS could therefore be a milder form of IBD.

▶ Question 8: Why are women more prone to IBS than men?

Doctors generally report three times as many female IBS patients as male. That's partly due to a greater male reluctance to consult a doctor about it. But even after allowing for that, it seems the incidence of IBS in women is double that in men. In one recent UK survey, 14.5 per cent of women had the symptoms but only 7 per cent of men. Why should this be? Here are five possible reasons:

▶ Dr Jeffrey Aron, Medical Director of the Center for Inflammatory Bowel Disorders at California Pacific Medical Center, believes the nerves that send signals from the gut to the brain are more developed in women than in men. As a result, any changes in gut function are more apparent to women and pain is more intense. He further believes the female brain processes gut signals in a different way, involving more areas that are linked to stress. Experiments show that women are certainly less tolerant of abdominal distension than men, suggesting that their guts are, indeed, more sensitive.

▶ Women have ovaries, a uterus and a vagina which may all compound the pain in the gut.

▶ Those who were sexually abused as children are more likely than others to develop an irritable bowel – and girls are more often abused than boys (see the entry on stress, below).

▶ 'Female' hormones seem to be implicated because about half to three-quarters of women with irritable bowels have worse symptoms during menstruation.

▶ Question 9: What does stress have to do with IBS?

Stress plays a role in many illnesses. It can be a very dangerous thing. In fact, many 'normal' people have digestive problems when they're under stress, not just irritable bowel sufferers. That's why we talk about 'scaring the shit' out of somebody.

Among other things, stress causes an increase in corticotrophin-releasing factor in the brain. As a result of that, activity in the stomach slows (to allow more energy to be diverted to the muscles) but activity in the lower digestive tract increases (to rid the body of the encumbrance of waste matter). Pain and diarrhoea may result.

Avoiding stress doesn't mean you have to keep away from everything that's exciting. The challenges you enjoy are good for you. It's the kind of stress that makes you feel anxious, overwhelmed or frightened that you need to avoid as far as possible.

As to whether or not stress can actually cause an irritable bowel, most doctors say it can't. But there is evidence that severe stress early in life, especially sexual abuse, can cause various physical problems later, including IBS. Women with abusive partners also tend to have a higher incidence of IBS.

However, IBS is not evidence of abuse and the majority of IBS sufferers were not abused.

▶ Question 10: What causes flare-ups?

IBS 'flares' may be caused by all sorts of things. The most common include:

- ▶ food you can't tolerate
- ▶ stress
- ▶ certain medicaments (especially antibiotics and antidepressants)
- ▶ anything containing sorbitol (a sweetener used in cough syrup and processed foods and which occurs naturally in some fruits)
- ▶ menstruation
- ▶ a change of oral contraceptives
- ▶ the bacterium C. *difficile*, which is carried by four to seven per cent of adults.

Case study

'One of the many frustrating aspects of IBS is getting other people to understand how serious it is and what it's like to be a sufferer. When they're a bit scornful or belittling I ask them to recall what it was like when they had the worst gastroenteritis of their lives. Then I ask them to imagine being in that condition every single day while commuting to work, trying to hold down a job, going shopping, or going out on a date. Then they begin to understand.' Diane (24)

The Seven Step Programme

Here, then, are the Seven Steps:

▶ Step 1: Understand your IBS

You're already well into Step 1. The more you know about irritable bowels, and the more you observe about your own circumstances, the more likely you are to identify the cause of your problems and to find a successful treatment, either on your own or together with your doctor, and with the help of this book. In the following chapters we'll be examining the remaining six steps in detail. Of course, it's quite possible that your particular problems may be solved in three steps or even by just one of the steps. But don't get despondent if you need all seven. That's the nature of the problem you're up against.

Try it now

Start an irritable bowel diary today recording everything you eat and drink, including medicines, everything you do, everything about the way you feel, and your bowel movements. Your diary will help you track down the cause of your problems and also be invaluable when you're discussing treatments with your doctor.

▶ Step 2: Get relief fast

You don't have to suffer without any relief while you're working your way through the Seven Step Programme. In your local high street or shopping mall there are things freely available that can make a huge difference to your condition. There are also some simple lifestyle changes you can easily make today. In Step 2 you'll learn all about them. If you can't wait, turn to Step 2 right now and find relief before the day is out.

▶ Step 3: Decide what you and your doctor are going to do

If you haven't yet seen a doctor it may be you feel discouraged by what you've read about the medical treatment of IBS. Perhaps you're embarrassed about the symptoms. Maybe you're someone who likes to solve problems on your own. But those are not good reasons. You need your doctor to rule out conditions other than IBS and, having done that, you then need to decide how much you're going to leave to your doctor and how much you're willing to do yourself.

Certain conditions can only be treated by a doctor, using medicines that (in most countries) are only available on prescription.

Doctors have quite an armoury of treatments that can help, including laxatives and fibre supplements to deal with constipation, tablets to stop diarrhoea, antispasmodics to prevent painful muscle spasms in the colon, antidepressants (especially tricyclic antidepressants) to reduce pain, antibiotics to kill 'bad' bacteria in the small intestine, and antiparasitics to kill intestinal parasites. You may decide to opt for every medicament advised, but even if you do there are still additional steps which only you can take.

So see a doctor but read this book in addition. No matter how much time doctors are willing to spend with you they're just not going to be able to convey all the information you need and that's in this book. And although a doctor can certainly recommend and supervise things like elimination diets, exercise programmes and stress reduction techniques, these kinds of things are largely down to you. This book will guide you through.

▶ Step 4: Take control of your diet

IBS means you can't handle certain foods. As we've seen, there can be a variety of reasons including SIBO, dysbiosis, enzyme deficiency, and a leaky gut. Step 4 is to identify the foods that trigger your symptoms and then to design a new way of eating. This is something very personal because what's good for someone else may not be good for you.

Key idea

You have ten times more microorganisms in your digestive tract than you have cells in your body. It's an astonishing thought. So it's really not surprising that the activities of those microorganisms should have a powerful impact on your gut as well as on your health generally.

▶ Step 5: Take control of your brains

Extraordinary as it may seem, your gut has its own 'brain', known as the 'enteric nervous system'. This 'brain' actually contains more neurons than the spinal cord – about 100 million. And many of the same neurotransmitters found in the central nervous system are also found in the gut, including serotonin, dopamine, noradrenaline (known as norepinephrine in the USA), glutamate and nitric oxide, along with neuropeptides, enkephalins (members of the 'feelgood' endorphin family) and even benzodiazepines (the family of chemicals of which valium is also a member).

Early in your development as a foetus there was a clump of tissue known as the 'neural crest'. That divided. One part formed your central nervous system while the other formed your enteric nervous system. Later, the two systems were linked by the vagus nerve. The vagus is also connected to the heart, as well as various other organs. The way all these parts of the body interact now starts to make sense.

It's not surprising that we use all kinds of phrases that reflect the special role of the gut. We say we have a 'gut instinct'. We say we can't 'stomach' something. We say we feel 'gutted'. We have 'butterflies in the tummy'. How accurate all these things are. Because our digestive tracts are closely linked with our emotions. There's even a new field of medicine called neurogastroenterology, entirely devoted to the interaction between the mind and the digestive system.

It's that interaction you'll be learning to control in Step 5.

Try it now

Here's an interesting little experiment. Think of something that frightens or worries you. It could be a violent and intimidating person, a huge drop from a skyscraper, a bill you can't pay, an exam you might fail, or something like that. Just spend a minute thinking about it and the consequences that might follow.

Done it? How do you feel? Tense? Head spinning a little? Mouth dry? What about your stomach? Do you have butterflies? A touch of heartburn? Stomach pain?

It's so common for your gut to respond to your emotions that you probably don't even question these kinds of reactions. But the fact that your gut can respond to your thoughts demonstrates how sensitive the mind-gut connection is.

▶ Step 6: Take control of your body

You may not feel much like exercising when you have irritable bowel symptoms but there's plenty of research to prove that it's an effective therapy. In a study by the University of Gothenburg, Sweden, half of a group of 102 IBS patients aged 18 to 65 were put on an exercise programme while the other half continued with their normal lives. Both groups received supportive calls from a physiotherapist but only the exercise group was encouraged to tackle 20 to 30 minutes of moderate to vigorous exercise three to five times a week. At the end of three months the results were astonishing. The symptoms of the non-exercise group had improved by only five points but for the exercise group the improvement was an impressive 51 points.

How does it work? Exercise massages the internal organs, helping to promote peristalsis in the gut, and releases trapped wind. It's also a proven way to increase endorphins and other painkilling, mood enhancing chemicals in the blood. In Step 6 we'll look at exercises that really help.

Try it now

Go for a short, brisk walk with plenty of arm swinging and from time to time when no one can see you jump up and down a bit. The idea is to assist the movement of the digestive tract and release some of that trapped gas.

▶ Step 7: Take control of your hormones

From various studies it's clear that about half to three-quarters of women with irritable bowels have worse symptoms during menstruation, particularly gas, abdominal pain and diarrhoea. So 'female' hormones are clearly implicated. High progesterone levels, for example, cause uterine cramping and in the same way they can also cause gastrointestinal cramping. But men can have hormone-related irritable bowel problems, too. In Step 7 you'll learn how to correct these hormonal problems.

Focus points

1 Irritable bowel syndrome (IBS) is a collection of symptoms affecting the intestines.
2 The symptoms include abdominal pain, bloating, and either constipation or diarrhoea or both alternately.
3 Beating IBS may require several different kinds of treatment.
4 The gut is a highly complicated organ with its own 'brain' and a huge and important population of microorganisms.
5 You will get better by following the Seven Steps.

In the next chapter

Sorting out all these different strands will take time. But, understandably, you don't want to wait. You want some relief right now. And you're going to have it. In Step 2 we'll be looking at some of the things you yourself can do immediately and in the next few hours. You won't be cured by them but you'll be able to live life in a more normal way while you're working on the Seven Step Programme.

2

Step 2: Get relief fast

In this chapter you will learn:

▶ *Techniques you can use right now at home to reduce or stop irritable bowel symptoms*

▶ *How strengthening your stomach acid could solve your problems*

▶ *How to prevent painful spasms and diarrhoea*

▶ *How to restore your gastrointestinal tract to health.*

Sorting out an irritable bowel can be a lengthy process. But there's no need to wait for relief. The suggestions in this chapter are certain to alleviate your symptoms within a few days, hours or even *minutes*. Depending on the cause or causes of your irritable bowel symptoms, some of them may amount to a cure. In other cases you should, at least, find they make life much, much more tolerable. All are worth trying.

Diagnostic test

Have you ever tried any of the following?

1 Enteric-coated peppermint oil capsules or other herbs, spices and minerals

2 Increasing stomach acidity with Betaine HCL/Apple Cider Vinegar (ACV)

3 Probiotic supplements

4 Enzyme supplements

5 Loperamide (Imodium™)

6 Heat

7 Squatting to defecate

8 Avoiding GI tract irritants

9 Relaxation and exercise

10 The pill (stopping or starting – women only).

Your score:

If you answered 'yes' to all of them you've obviously been struggling with an irritable bowel for a long time but there may still be some quick remedies you've missed. If you answered 'yes' to just a few questions you have useful things to discover. If you answered 'no' to most or all questions there are things in this chapter that could dramatically change your life.

Take enteric-coated peppermint oil capsules

Enteric-coated peppermint oil capsules (that's to say, they dissolve in the small intestine, not in the stomach) are the number-one fast self-treatment for irritable bowels, especially IBS-D. Don't dismiss them as some kind of herbal mumbo jumbo. Peppermint is scientifically recognized as a powerful antispasmodic and is often prescribed by doctors. And, in fact, in at least one review, enteric-coated peppermint oil capsules performed better than any other IBS medicament, having a Number Needed To Treat (NNT) of just 2.5. That's exceptional. (For an explanation of NNT see the Key idea below.)

A study by the Department of Internal Medicine at Taichung Veterans General Hospital in Taiwan compared an enteric-coated peppermint-oil formulation (Colpermin) with a placebo for the treatment of IBS. In more than half of cases the peppermint provided complete pain relief and in four-fifths of sufferers it provided at least some. It was also very successful against diarrhoea, bloating and flatulence. These were the full results:

	Enteric-coated peppermint oil	Placebo
Percentage that experienced:		
Reduced pain	79	43
Of which, complete pain relief	56	8
Reduced abdominal distension	83	29
Reduced stool frequency	83	32
Fewer borborygmi (stomach rumbles)	73	31
Less flatulence	79	22

How does peppermint work? Because it's an anti-spasmodic, peppermint calms the smooth muscles of the stomach and intestines. It also has analgesic (painkilling) properties.

Researchers at the University of Adelaide, Australia, have found that it acts through an 'anti-pain' channel called TRPM8. For some irritable bowel sufferers, peppermint is almost magical, completely relieving pain and reducing other symptoms, too. For the lucky ones it's virtually an instant 'cure' and a substantial majority enjoy at least some benefit.

However, there is a problem with enteric-coated peppermint if you have IBS-C. By reducing the activity of the intestinal muscles, it will probably make constipation worse.

▶ Why do I need enteric coating?

Both 'extra strong' mints and mint tea will also bring some relief. The problem with them is that they not only relax the muscles of the gut but also the lower oesophageal sphincter. That potentially allows stomach acid to splash up into the oesophagus (the tube down which food enters the stomach) causing the painful burning sensation known as heartburn. That's where the 'enteric-coating' comes in. Because the capsules pass through the stomach undigested, only releasing the peppermint oil once they get to the small intestine, the peppermint can't influence the lower oesophageal sphincter.

You can find these enteric-coated capsules in chemists and health food stores. Think of peppermint tea and peppermints only as a stop-gap and get the enteric-coated capsules as soon as possible.

Remember this

Enteric-coated peppermint oil capsules must be swallowed whole, not chewed. It's best to take them on an empty stomach with the minimum of water and to wait a while before eating or drinking anything else. First thing in the morning is a good time. If you're also taking medication to lower stomach acid, have the peppermint capsules first and the indigestion medication at least an hour later (but see below about *increasing* stomach acid).

Key idea

A Number Needed to Treat (NNT) is a measure used by doctors and scientists to work out how effective a treatment is. It's defined as the number of patients you need to treat to prevent one additional bad outcome. For example, an NNT of five for a medicament would mean that out of every five patients treated there would be one more who recovered than if none had been treated. The key point to bear in mind is that the higher the number the less effective the treatment and the lower the number the more effective the treatment. Note that different studies may arrive at different NNTs.

Case study

'I've had IBS for about 25 years. Initially I would have a flare up a couple of times a year but recently it started to be a couple of times a month. When I had a flare up the pain was so severe that I would black out in the toilet. As a result I've had a broken nose and a broken rib. About three months ago I started taking one enteric-coated peppermint oil capsule every night before going to bed and I've not had any IBS symptoms at all since then. Nothing! I'd recommend anybody with IBS to try these.' Alan (55)

Other herbs, spices and minerals

Enteric-coated peppermint oil is definitely the top herb/spice/mineral for irritable bowels (especially IBS-D). But there are others that are certainly worth considering.

Ginger (*Zingiber officinale*) has been used in China for more than 2,000 years to treat digestive problems. Here are just some of the things it can do:

► Reduce wind, according to researchers at India's G.B. Pant University.

► Calm spasms in the digestive tract, according to researchers at the Aga Khan University Medical College in Pakistan.

- Speed gastric emptying, according to a study published in the *World Journal of Gastroenterology*.

- Combat fungal infections, according to the Biology Department of Carleton University, Canada.

- Treat bacterial diarrhoea, according to researchers at the China Medical University in Taichung.

- Inhibit stomach ulcers, according to a study by the Kyoto Pharmaceutical University, Japan.

- Relieve menstrual pain. Researchers at the Nursing and Midwifery School in Tehran, Iran, found ginger as effective for this as ibuprofen. This makes ginger particularly useful when irritable bowel symptoms are exacerbated by period pains.

- Combat nausea. In a study at the University of Rochester Medical Center, headed by Julie L. Ryan, those who took ginger supplements along with standard anti-vomiting drugs suffered 40 per cent less nausea following chemotherapy. (The ginger was given for three days prior to the treatment and for three days afterwards.) Even more impressive, ginger performed better than the motion-sickness drug Dramamine® in volunteers who sat in a spinning tilted chair.

- Reduce inflammation (and, therefore, the pain that goes with it). And ginger does it more safely than non-steroidal anti-inflammatory drugs (NSAIDs), such as ibuprofen. NSAIDs inhibit an enzyme known as COX-2 (thus reducing inflammation) but also COX-1, which normally protects the stomach. The result is that NSAIDs can damage the stomach and cause bleeding. Ginger is extremely cunning. One of its actions is to block COX-2 but not COX-1, something that medical science has only recently achieved with the painkiller celecoxib. But while man-made COX-2-only inhibitors have serious side-effects, ginger has almost none. Comparing ginger and NSAIDs in terms of pain control, one study found that, when used over a period of weeks, ginger was as effective as ibuprofen at reducing the joint pain caused by osteoarthritis. In another study, ginger provided significant pain relief to more than three-quarters of those who suffered from rheumatoid arthritis or osteoarthritis.

▶ Thin the blood, according to Dr K Srivastava at the Institute of Community Health in Odense, Denmark.

▶ Kill cancer cells in the laboratory, according to various research studies, including one by the University of Michigan Comprehensive Cancer Center.

▶ Help in the management of diabetes, according to a study by the Faculty of Science at Kuwait University.

▶ How should I use ginger?

If you're using fresh ginger you can simply peel a little of the rhizome and chew on it. You can also cut half a dozen thin slices from the rhizome to make an infusion with boiling water. In the form of tablets, up to around 500 mg of extract per day should be fine.

▶ Does ginger have any side-effects?

The United States Food and Drug Administration (FDA) says ginger is 'generally recognized as safe' but there are a few provisos. Some people are allergic to ginger and there have been cases in which it caused arrhythmia (irregular heartbeat). At doses above 500 mg per day it may increase blood pressure. Because ginger has slight blood thinning properties it shouldn't be used with anticoagulants. Don't take ginger with NSAIDs or diabetic medicines.

More alternatives

▶ **Anise (also known as aniseed).** An infusion of the ground seeds in boiling water relieves wind and constipation. Note that as anise is a laxative you should avoid it if you suffer from IBS-D.

▶ **Calcium supplements.** Some IBS-D sufferers find calcium stops diarrhoea when other remedies have failed. In one study at St Luke's/Roosevelt Hospital Center, New York, either 2400 or 3600 mg of calcium carbonate per day were given to intestinal bypass patients over a period of 12 weeks. Bowel frequency was reduced by 49 per cent and stools were significantly less watery. However, this is a high dose and should not be continued for a long time due to the risk of calcium becoming deposited in the arteries. Many users report that calcium works best when taken at the end of every meal.

▶ **Chamomile**. An infusion of the flowers reduces gastrointestinal inflammation and is both an antibacterial and an antispasmodic.

▶ **Fennel**. An infusion of the dried seeds eases bloating, heartburn and spasms in the large intestine. It has a pleasant liquorice flavour.

▶ **Liquorice**. In one study carried out by Goulds Naturopathica in Hobart, Australia, a mixture of liquorice root, slippery elm (see below), lactulose and oat bran improved bowel habit and symptoms in patients with IBS-C. Liquorice has been in use as a medicinal herb for over 3,000 years and is now known to protect the stomach from acid by increasing the formation of new mucosal cells and by stimulating them to produce more mucin. The glycyrrhizin in liquorice can cause high blood pressure and oedema, so it's recommended to buy it in the form of chewable deglycyrrhizinated tablets (known as DGL liquorice).

▶ **Magnesium**. An important mineral, it's involved in many bodily processes. But most Westerners consume below the RDA (recommended daily amount or recommended dietary allowance). As regards irritable bowels, magnesium has the property of relaxing the muscles of the gastrointestinal tract, thus easing painful spasms and encouraging steady movement of food through the system. It also attracts water into the intestines, softening the stool and making everything more slippery. Foods high in magnesium include nuts, seeds, whole grains and legumes. If you eat them regularly you'll have enough magnesium. If not a supplement of 200–300 mg a day would be good for your health and your IBS-C.

- **Slippery elm.** Slippery elm (*Ulmus fulva*) is a North American tree long used by Native Americans to treat a variety of problems. Dried and powdered, the inner bark has the ability to stimulate mucous secretion in the gut, thus combating inflammation. It makes a nice drink added to, say, oat milk, or can be taken in capsules. (Only add it to cow's milk if you're certain you're not lactose intolerant.)

- **Turmeric.** Often known as 'Indian saffron' this spice has a deep yellow colour and is used in curries. It's a powerful anti-inflammatory and combats flatulence and stomach pain, as well as having various other benefits.

- **Wild yam.** Sold under various names including wild Mexican yam, colic root and rheumatism root, this herb is both an antispasmodic and an anti-inflammatory. Some irritable bowel sufferers say their symptoms have been completely alleviated by taking wild yam in capsule or powder form every morning.

Increase your stomach acid

If you ever get heartburn you probably imagine your stomach acid is too strong. But, very often, the reverse is the case. Weak stomach acid can not only be a cause of heartburn but also irritable bowel symptoms. It's a common disorder, especially among the middle aged or older, and it's very easily fixed. Here are just some of the problems associated with it:

- Heartburn

- Stomach pains

- Bloating

- Diarrhoea

- A tender feeling around the stomach area

- Bacterial overgrowth

- Susceptibility to food poisoning

- Poor absorption of protein

- Poor absorption of electrolytes such as zinc and magnesium

- Poor absorption of vitamins, especially B complex, C and K

- Food allergies.

You may be asking how a burning sensation in your oesophagus can be caused by *weak* stomach acid. Surely it must be too strong? Isn't that why people take antacids? Here's the explanation for the paradox. Acid is kept out of your oesophagus by the lower oesophageal sphincter. That sphincter (valve) requires strong acid in the stomach if it's to remain tightly closed (except, of course, for the passage of food and drink). If stomach acid is too weak the valve may stay a little open. It's then that acid can splash up into the oesophagus, especially when you bend over or lie down in bed. Unlike the stomach itself, the oesophagus has no protection against acid so those splashes hurt (even if the acid is weaker than it should be).

So weak stomach acid could be contributing to your irritable bowel symptoms or it could even be the entire explanation. In addition you may be suffering food allergies because pepsin, an enzyme that breaks down protein in the stomach, only functions properly in strong acid. If pepsin doesn't go to work as it should, large proteins can pass through the gut wall triggering an immune (allergic) response.

How will you know if your stomach acid is weak? The best thing is to get your doctor to run a test (see Step 3). The pH of the stomach is normally between one and five, depending on whether it's empty or full, and what you've been eating. The lower the number the stronger the acid. Seven is neutral and anything above seven is alkaline (basic). In the meantime, there are two home tests you can try right away.

Remember this

It's thought that in adulthood the strength of stomach acid declines by around one percentage point a year and that in at least half of those aged over 60 it's significantly low. So if you're no longer young it's unlikely you have stomach acid that's too strong or too copious.

Try it now

Here's the first test, using something you probably have in the kitchen:

1 Upon waking, before drinking or eating, mix a ¼ teaspoon of baking soda in a glass of water and drink it.
2 Time how long it takes before you belch:
  ▷ Within the first four minutes – acid level okay
  ▷ After four to ten minutes – low acid
  ▷ Longer than ten minutes – very low acid.

Try it now

The baking soda test is rather crude so use it only as a guide. A better home test uses Betaine HCL tablets. HCL stands for hydrochloric acid, which is the acid you have in your stomach. Taking the tablet will give it a boost (so don't do this if you have ulcers):

1 Purchase Betaine HCL tablets (available from health shops).
2 Take one tablet in the middle of a meal.
3 After half an hour or so:
  ▷ If you notice a warm sensation (as if you'd swallowed strong alcohol on an empty stomach) then your stomach acid level is probably okay.
  ▷ If you notice nothing (that is, the combination of the tablet and your stomach acid wasn't enough to create a warm sensation) then your stomach acid is probably too weak.

Again, the Betaine HCL test is rather crude and it's always possible that the warm or burning sensation is caused by a damaged mucosal barrier rather than acid that's been made unnaturally strong. So a doctor's confirmation is important.

▶ What's the solution?

If you conclude that you do have weak stomach acid, how can you correct it? Here are two ways:

▶ Take Betaine HCL with meals.

▶ Take apple cider vinegar (ACV) with meals.

The strength of Betaine HCL tablets varies according to the manufacturer, but most are around 650–1000 mg. Usually the tablets also contain the enzyme pepsin, which breaks down protein.

The idea is to build up the number of tablets until you get a warm sensation in your stomach. Then for all subsequent meals you take one less than that number of tablets. If the warm sensation actually becomes painful sip a glass of water into which ¼ teaspoon of baking soda has been dissolved (and don't take that number of tablets again). So your programme might go like this:

▶ **Meal 1**. Take one tablet. No feeling of warmth.

▶ **Meal 2**. Take two tablets. A hint of warmth.

▶ **Meal 3**. Take three tablets. Definite feeling of warmth.

▶ **All subsequent meals**. Take two tablets.

An alternative to Betaine HCL is apple cider vinegar (ACV). It has a pH of 3 but as it needs to be diluted in water its effective pH is higher (that is, the acid is weaker). Most nutritionists recommend organic, unfiltered, unpasteurized ACV that contains the 'mother' (that is, it looks cloudy).

Incidentally, ACV has been shown to lower blood glucose levels, and therefore protect against Type 2 diabetes, reduce the risk of oesophageal cancer, and help with diarrhoea, so it has additional benefits. On the down side, one study found an increased risk of bladder cancer.

Start with about three good teaspoonfuls in a small glass of water with every meal and then adjust the dose according to the results. Given the rather sour taste you may prefer to switch to Betaine HCL.

▶ **What do I do if I'm taking proton-pump inhibitors/histamine type 2 receptor blockers to reduce stomach acid?**

If you suffer from heartburn, gastroesophageal reflux disease (GERD) or ulcers it may well be that you're taking either proton-pump inhibitors (such as omeprazole) or histamine type 2 receptor blockers (such as cimetidine) to reduce stomach acid. If you're prescribed them for ulcers then you should not take Betaine HCL or ACV. However, if you're taking them for heartburn or GERD, you should consider giving those medicines up and then *increasing* your stomach acid as described. Discuss this with your doctor.

Key idea

If you've been taking proton-pump inhibitors or histamine type 2 receptor blockers for a while, your pain on giving them up may even be worse than it was before you started the medicine. Naturally you see the pain as confirmation that the medicine is essential, but it may not be. The pain is all to do with what's known as the 'rebound' effect. The solution is to taper off slowly by gradually reducing the dose over a month. (You can open the capsules and take only, say, three-quarters of the contents, then half, then a quarter.) Once you're off the capsules you can move on to the Betaine HCL or ACV.

Remember this

Betaine HCL tablets should be swallowed straight down without chewing. Don't take them if you have ulcers.

Take probiotics but not prebiotics

As we saw in Step 1, there are 'good' and 'bad' bacteria in your gut. The 'bad' can cause irritable bowel symptoms but are kept down by the 'good' (which also confer health benefits). Problems arise if the colonies of 'good' bacteria come under attack from something such as antibiotics, or if additional 'bad' bacteria are imported on contaminated food. Then the 'bad' bacteria get the upper hand. An obvious way to combat them is to import more of the 'good' bacteria in the form of probiotics.

Probiotics are defined as live microorganisms which when administered in adequate amounts confer a health benefit on the host. They come naturally with certain foods but they can also be taken as supplements. We'll be looking at food in Step 4. Here we'll be concentrating on the supplements.

The theory of probiotic supplements is completely logical. But does it work in practice? Probiotic supplements are measured in terms of colony forming units (CFUs). The recommended level is 10 billion CFUs as the minimum effective dose (MED). Not all supplements contain that level. Even those that do at the time of manufacture may not at the time of purchase. Remember, the bacteria need to be alive when you swallow the capsules. ConsumerLab.com surveyed various probiotic supplements and found that at the time of purchase they contained from 58 per cent to as little as 10 per cent of the amount of bacteria listed on the label. After they've been stored at home for a while the live content would be even less.

The second hurdle is that probiotics have to survive the acid environment of the stomach before they can get to work in the small and large intestines. Experiments suggest that many of them don't.

The third hurdle is simply to do with the limits of current scientific knowledge. There are hundreds of strains of bacteria in the intestines and scientists as yet have very little data on which ones work for IBS and which make symptoms worse.

That having been said, there are very strong arguments for giving probiotic supplements a try.

Take the bacteria known as *Lactobacillus plantarum*, for example. (All bacteria have rather intimidating Latin names, but don't let that put you off.) There's evidence that it's capable of withstanding stomach acid as well as bile acids and of colonizing the gastrointestinal tract, if only temporarily. At the same time, it seems the population of high gas-producing bacteria such as *Veillonella* and *Clostridia* declines in the presence of *Lactobacillus plantarum*.

Does it do any good? The *Lactobacillus plantarum* strain Lp299v was tested on IBS sufferers by Professor Philippe Ducrotté from Rouen University Hospital, France, and found to reduce abdominal pain and bloating. That strain is available as a supplement.

Another interesting candidate is *Bifidobacterium infantis 35624* (available under the brand name Bifantis). In 2006, it was studied by a team under Dr Peter Whorwell, Professor of Medicine and Gastroenterology at the University of Manchester. They gave *Bifidobacterium infantis 35624* to a group of women aged 18 to 65 once a day for four weeks. At the end of the month there was significant improvement in their IBS symptoms and, as a bonus, the bacteria appeared to reduce inflammation, opening up a possible treatment for diseases such as arthritis.

Both *Bifidobacterium infantis* and *Lactobacillus plantarum* are in a probiotic 'medical food' called VSL#3 which is manufactured in the USA and marketed worldwide. In addition VSL#3 contains live lyophilized (frozen and dehydrated) *Bifidobacterium breve, Bifidobacterium longum, Lactobacillus acidophilus, Lactobacillus paracasei, Lactobacillus bulgaricus* and *Streptococcus thermophilus*. In one study (Selinger CP, Bell A, Cairns A, Lockett M, Sebastian S, Haslam N) VSL#3 prevented diarrhoea induced by antibiotics. In another (Dharmani P, De Simone C, Chadee K) VSL#3 accelerated gastric ulcer healing by stimulating vascular endothelial growth factor – that's to say, by encouraging the renewal of the stomach lining. It's also been shown to have anti-inflammatory effects.

Anecdotal evidence is also overwhelmingly positive on IBS forums.

So VSL#3 is looking very promising. But here's something very curious. Although in yet another study (Michail S, Kenche H) VSL#3 was shown to have a positive effect on diarrhoea, the researchers found no change in gut microbiota. They concluded there must have been a different mechanism of action. So there's still a long way to go on probiotic research.

Reviewing all the serious studies that have been done so far it can be said that probiotics:

- enhance gut barrier function (reduce 'leaky gut')
- reduce inflammation
- reduce pain
- reduce flatulence and bloating.

Key idea

VSL#3 is quite expensive, especially by mail order (because of the need for insulated boxes and couriers). Many irritable bowel sufferers find they can make it more economical by using just half a sachet at a time or even a quarter (which still contains more than 100 billion bacteria).

Remember this

When you're buying probiotic supplements for an irritable bowel:

► Make sure each dose contains at least 10 billion CFUs.
► Buy only from a source that has a fast turnover (ask how long the product has been in stock – most probiotics shouldn't be stored at room temperature for more than a month following manufacture).
► At home, store the supplement in the fridge, unless instructed otherwise.

As an alternative to capsules and powders it's possible to buy foods deliberately made with, or enhanced with, 'good' bacteria. Activia probiotic yoghurt is an example. A controlled trial published in the journal *Alimentary Pharmacology and Therapeutics* (Guyonnet D *et al*), found that women with IBS-C who ate two pots of Activia a day had increased stool frequency, less bloating and a better quality of life. Activia contains *Bifidobacterium lactis* (which the manufacturers, Danone, call *Bifidus ActiRegularis*).

PREBIOTIC SUPPLEMENTS – NOT A GOOD IDEA, YET

Bacteria in the gut feed on prebiotics, which are a small but natural part of most people's diets (they're in bananas, onions and whole wheat, for example). If you have a healthy gut then taking a prebiotic supplement to give the bacteria a boost can be a good idea. But if you have irritable bowel symptoms you may simply be feeding 'bad' bacteria and making your situation worse. Fructooligosaccharides (FOS), for example, are a type of prebiotic that can cause gas, bloating, intestinal cramps and diarrhoea in some people. Galactooligosaccharides (GOS) can be a better bet because the 'good' bacteria usually get to them first. You'll find GOS in certain processed foods. But as a general rule you need to get the balance of your bacteria right before you deliberately feed them additional prebiotics.

We'll be looking at natural prebiotics and their effects in Step 4.

Take enzyme supplements

Enzymes are catalysts, that's to say, they speed up metabolic reactions, including the digestion of food, by millions of times. Each type of food requires its own enzyme or enzymes and if, for whatever reason, you're deficient then the nutrients won't be absorbed by you. Instead the food will pass along to the large intestine where it will make a banquet for the bacteria there. Gas, bloating and pain will be the result.

Supplements seem to be the obvious solution to a deficiency. In theory all you have to do is take them with a meal and they'll work on that actual meal, providing a more or less instant remedy. Assuming, that is, they work at all. The fact is, oral enzyme supplements are controversial. Many experts say they're deactivated by stomach acid and can't work. Well-designed studies to try to settle the issue have been quite rare. So let's see what we do know:

▶ Different enzymes need different levels of acidity. Gastric lipase, for example, needs low acidity of pH 5 or 6. By contrast, pepsin, which breaks up proteins in the stomach, is most effective in strong acid with a pH of 2. So a pepsin supplement, for one, should certainly work.

▶ Dr Edward Howell (1898–1988) was a pioneer of enzyme supplementation and wrote two books on the subject. From his clinical experience he was convinced that they work. His recommendation was to open the capsules and sprinkle the contents on food, to begin the process of digestion as early as possible.

▶ Researchers at the Gastroenterology Unit of the University of Salerno, Italy, gave Biointol®, a commercial enzyme preparation, to 50 IBS patients and concluded that it significantly reduced bloating, flatulence and abdominal pain. In another study, IBS-D sufferers were given lipase to take before any high-fat meal. The researchers concluded it reduced cramping, bloating, pain and urgency.

▶ People suffering from pancreatic exocrine insufficiency are successfully treated with oral pancrelipase containing lipase, protease and amylase (see Step 3).

▶ The enzyme alpha-galactosidase helps break down complex sugars as found in beans, peas, lentils, cauliflower, broccoli and cabbage. A 2007 study published in *Digestive Diseases and Sciences* found that an alpha-galactosidase supplement cut the average number of flatulent episodes following bean meals from 16 to 10 with a standard dose and to just five with four-times the standard dose.

▶ In Britain, the National Health Service (NHS) rates an oral lactase substitute as 'very effective' for those who, for whatever reason, do not produce sufficient lactase themselves. Dosing is very much a question of trial and error but start with 6,000–9,000 IU after the first few bites of a meal that contains dairy so that the food provides some protection from stomach acid. Don't take the supplement late in the meal as it might then be too late to make a difference.

In the absence of really good scientific trials it's impossible to make a definitive statement. But the experimental and anecdotal evidence to say that oral enzyme supplements are beneficial for some irritable bowel sufferers is persuasive. Compared to the enzymes that occur naturally in food, supplements are extremely potent and could still have an effect even if a large proportion of the enzymes are 'denatured' in the stomach. Certainly they're worth a try. You'll find more on natural enzymes in Step 4.

Key idea

It pays to shop around for enzymes, both in terms of the price and in terms of their effectiveness for you. The most expensive is not necessarily the best. If the first brand you try doesn't work in your case try at least two more before giving up on them.

> **Remember this**
>
> Enzymes do not build up in the body. If your body doesn't produce enough enzymes you'll have to take them with every meal and snack.

Take loperamide or kaolin and morphine for IBS-D

Loperamide, sold under various brand names including Imodium™, is an opioid that reduces or stops diarrhoea. It works by decreasing the tone of the longitudinal smooth muscles while increasing the tone of the circular smooth muscles, thus increasing the amount of time waste matter remains in the large intestine. That in turn leads to more water being absorbed from the faecal matter. So loperamide is a useful medicament for flare-ups of IBS-D, especially when you're, say, travelling or have social engagements.

Note that in some cases loperamide can actually cause abdominal pain and bloating as well as nausea and, in rare cases, dizziness. It should not be given to children under two years of age.

Kaolin and morphine is a mixture that has been in use for many years. Kaolin is an absorbent that helps rid the gut of toxins, while the morphine slows the passage of waste through the large intestine allowing more water to be removed. As a result stools are firmer and it's not necessary to go to the toilet so often. The standard dose is 10ml every four hours during attacks of diarrhoea.

Note that kaolin and morphine should not be taken regularly as a preventive measure because the morphine content is potentially addictive. Kaolin and morphine may interact with the kinds of antidepressants known as monoamine oxidase inhibitors (MAOIs) as well as sedatives and sleeping pills. Side-effects may include nausea, drowsiness, facial flushing, dry mouth, sweating and constipation. Consult your doctor before taking this medicine if you are pregnant, trying to become pregnant, or breastfeeding.

Apply heat

Everyone knows that a hot water bottle on the stomach is comforting and relaxes tense muscles. But science has now proven that your favourite hot water bottle can actually deactivate pain at the molecular level, in much the same way as painkilling tablets. The mechanism is this.

If heat over 40° C is applied to the skin over the site of internal pain, heat receptors (known as TRPV1) are switched on, which in turn block pain receptors (known as P2X3) that cause the perception of pain. Research continues into a drug that will block P2X3 but in the meantime heat is a satisfactory method in many cases.

Dr Brian King at the Department of Physiology, University College London, who has led research into heat, says it's particularly effective for short-term pain relief for the body's hollow organs. In a speech to the Physiological Society he said that the pain of colic (inflammation and distension of the GI tract) 'is caused by a temporary reduction in blood flow to or over-distension of hollow organs such as the bowel or uterus, causing local tissue damage and activating pain receptors.' Heat helps to restore the blood flow.

There are various ways of applying heat:

▶ **Hot water bottles**. In the sixteenth century, metal bed warmers were filled with hot coals from the fire and used to warm the sheets before getting in. Quite soon someone had the idea of using containers of hot water which could safely be kept in the bed. Initially they were made of glass, earthenware, zinc, copper and even wood until the hot water bottle as we know it was invented by the Croatian engineer Slavoljub Penkala (1871–1922).

▶ **Microwave heating pads**. These contain a gel and can be heated in a microwave oven.

▶ **Chemical pads**. Hot water bottles and microwave pads are cumbersome. Chemical pads have the advantage that they can be stuck to the body and be invisible under clothes. Generally they contain reagents which, when the pad is squeezed hard enough, mix and create heat lasting eight to ten hours. Their disadvantage is that they're expensive and can be used only once. However, there are reusable versions containing a supersaturated solution of sodium acetate.

▶ **Electric pads.** These are mostly used by professional therapists. It would only be worth buying one for home use if your irritable bowel pain is frequent and severe.

▶ **Infrared lamps.** Good as surface heating can be, it's limited by the fact that the temperature of the heat device shouldn't exceed more than about 42° C, the heat being transferred from the surface of the skin to the lower levels by conduction. One method of getting the heat more directly where it's needed is to use infrared radiation. The sensation is very much like lying in the sun. Note that IR-B and IR-C rays have very little penetration – for a useful effect you need IR-A.

▶ **Saunas and steam rooms.** Most people's perception is that wet heat (as in a steam room) gets into the body faster. However, research by Regina M Fink RN clearly showed that dry heat (as in a sauna) was more effective at causing vasodilation, one of the key benefits of heat therapy. Saunas also have the advantage of reducing muscle stiffness and fatigue.

Obviously the relief only lasts during the time that you're applying the heat. But a good old-fashioned hot water bottle can help you get through a crisis.

Remember this

Don't apply heat to your stomach area if, for any reason, it's bruised or swollen, or you've recently had abdominal surgery.

Become a squatter

According to some experts, a huge number of digestive tract problems are caused or exacerbated by nothing more than the modern toilet. Although there's not much scientific evidence there's an undeniable scientific logic about it. The fact is, human beings are designed to squat not sit. And, indeed, in those parts of the world where the Western toilet is a rarity so too are many of the Western world's digestive system disorders.

Here, according to 'squatters', is the full list of problems caused or exacerbated by the modern toilet:

- Appendicitis
- Bladder incontinence
- Colitis
- Crohn's disease
- Colon cancer
- Constipation
- Diverticulitis
- Fainting on the toilet
- Gastroesophageal reflux disease (GERD)
- Gynaecological problems

- Heart attacks
- Haemorrhoids
- Hiatus Hernia
- Incomplete emptying of the rectum
- Prostate problems
- Sexual dysfunction
- Small Intestinal Bacterial Overgrowth (SIBO)
- Strokes.

As an irritable bowel sufferer you'll be especially interested in two items on the list, firstly that sensation of incomplete emptying of the rectum and, secondly, the condition known as small intestinal bacterial overgrowth (SIBO), which many doctors think is the prime cause of irritable bowel symptoms. But you wouldn't want to have any of the problems on the list if you could avoid them.

There are two reasons it can feel as if the rectum didn't empty completely. One is that the rectum continues to contract for a time, even though there's nothing in it. That can be quite uncomfortable and even painful. The second reason, quite simply, is that evacuation *is* incomplete.

The fact is that when you sit, your puborectalis muscle constricts the area where the rectum joins the anal canal, making it more difficult to defecate. When you squat, by contrast, the puborectalis relaxes, leaving a clear passage for waste. In addition, the thighs give support to the colon. The result should be complete and strain-free evacuation.

Squatting has another huge advantage for irritable bowel sufferers. When you go to the toilet in the sitting position, significant pressure is exerted on the ileocecal (IC) valve. The job of the IC is to prevent bacteria-laden waste backing up from the large intestine into the small intestine. If the IC leaks, bacteria from the large intestine, where they're needed, get into the small intestine, where they shouldn't be. The result is small intestinal bacterial overgrowth (SIBO). Doctors argue about the true prevalence of SIBO, but one thing is clear. When you have SIBO you also have irritable bowel symptoms. SIBO is discussed in detail in Step 4.

One of the stories of Catherine the Great (1729–1796), Empress of Russia, is that her death at the age of 67 was caused by a stroke brought on by straining on the toilet. The stroke is a fact and the toilet aspect is certainly plausible because the sit toilet often requires the use of the 'Valsalva Manoeuvre'. That's to say, you hold your breath and push down with the diaphragm. This aids defecation but increases pressure within the thoracic cavity, reducing the flow of blood to the heart. The result can be fainting or even a stroke or heart attack. Squatting reduces the need for the Valsalva Manoeuvre. Other famous people who probably died in this way include Elvis Presley and George II of Great Britain.

Remember this

Do your abdominal muscles seem to 'collapse' for a time after defecation, causing your stomach to look bloated? That's a sign the muscles have been straining too much.

Try it now

Next time you need to defecate, and assuming you're agile enough and not too heavy for your normal toilet, try squatting on the toilet seat. Otherwise you can buy frames that create a strong platform around the toilet, or you could replace your existing toilet with a proper squat toilet.

Note that placing a stool in front of the toilet to raise the feet in an approximation of the squatting position is not effective, nor is adopting the 'ski' position. The essence of the true squatting position is that all the weight is taken on the feet, with the buttocks more or less between the ankles. It can seem difficult at first but try a few times before deciding if it's for you. The key is to hug your thighs against your abdomen and use that pressure, rather than your diaphragm, to help things along.

Remember this

The squatting position is not an automatic cure for straining. In fact, because it's not very comfortable you might be tempted to hurry things up using excessive pressure from your abdominal muscles and diaphragm, just as when sitting. That defeats the whole object. The important thing, whether squatting or sitting, is to be relaxed. Don't go to the bathroom before you need to. There are stretch receptors in the rectum which will initiate contractions when the rectum is sufficiently full. There's no point trying to squeeze waste matter out of an insufficiently full rectum by conscious force. Wait until you feel the contractions of the rectal muscles, then go to the bathroom and allow them to do their work.

Eliminate GI tract irritants

Identifying the food and drink that's upsetting you can be a complicated process. We'll be tackling that in Step 4. But certain foods, drink (and medicines) are well known to irritate the gastrointestinal tract in sensitive individuals. So it would make sense for you to cut down on or even entirely avoid the following *as from now*, if possible:

► Alcohol. Researchers led by Scott Gabbard MD at the Dartmouth-Hitchcock Medical Center and the Mayo Clinic have shown a clear link between even moderate alcohol consumption and SIBO. 'Moderate' was defined as one drink a day for women or two drinks a day for men.

► Caffeine

► Carbonated drinks

► Chocolate

- Coffee including decaffeinated coffee. As little as one cup of coffee stimulates muscle contractions in the large intestine and rectum in sensitive individuals

- Fatty food

- Ibuprofen and other non-steroidal anti-inflammatory drugs (NSAIDs)

- Milk and dairy products, unless you're certain you're not lactose intolerant

- Sorbitol.

Relaxation and exercise

There's no doubt that irritable bowel symptoms are exacerbated by stress. Even people who have normal digestion can suffer from diarrhoea when anxious or scared. So combating stress is a treatment for an irritable bowel and exercise is one way of doing it. Exercise increases production of endorphins, the body's own natural painkillers and mood boosters.

We'll be looking at some highly effective relaxation techniques in Step 5 and some exercise ideas in Step 6. Right now I'm going to show you a relaxation technique which is highly effective and which you can put into action straight away. All you have to do is modify the way you breathe.

It works like this. When you're frightened (let's say, by a dangerous animal) your breathing becomes very shallow and constricted. Without deliberately intending to, you may even hold your breath entirely. It's a natural and logical response because it makes you less obvious to the predator that's stalking you. Conversely, when you're feeling very relaxed your breathing will naturally be slow.

Here's the clever bit. Rather than letting your autonomic nervous system decide how you'll breathe, you can take conscious charge of your breathing. By doing so you turn everything back to front. You force your body to enter the state that corresponds with the way you've chosen to breathe. In other words, if you consciously make your breathing deep and slow with longer exhalations than inhalations, you actually compel your body to relax, even if you're in a dangerous situation. It can't do otherwise.

Here's how it's done:

- ▶ Place a hand on your stomach and breathe in through your nose so your belly rises but your chest and shoulders hardly move at all.

- ▶ Aim to expand your stomach to the maximum during a count of seven.

- ▶ Hold your breath for a count of two.

- ▶ With your hand still in place, breathe out through your mouth for a count of 11, all the time feeling your stomach go down.

- ▶ Wait for a count of two then breathe in again for a count of seven.

- ▶ Continue like this (7 – 2 – 11 – 2 – 7 – 2 – 11 ...) for ten cycles (or longer if you wish).

Nothing too strenuous about that. It's something you should be doing every day, whenever you feel under pressure or anxious. And you should also be aiming for some physical exercise every day as well. We'll be seeing how that works later in the book. For the moment just keep in mind that exercise helps reduce irritable bowel symptoms by:

- ▶ encouraging the release of trapped wind

- ▶ restoring normal peristalsis in the digestive tract

- ▶ releasing the body's own mood-boosting and pain-killing chemicals known as endorphins.

So if you're not already exercising regularly, start today (in a way suitable for your age and state of health).

Start/stop the pill

Many women report their irritable bowel symptoms started when they went on the pill. Sometimes switching to a different type of pill helps, sometimes it doesn't. Others say they already had IBS and that going on the pill actually reduced symptoms. Still others say they never had IBS until they stopped taking the pill. The only thing that's clear is that there's some kind of connection between menstrual cycles, birth control pills and irritable bowels and the common factor has to be hormones (and men can have hormone-related irritable bowel symptoms, too).

Generally, it's desirable to maintain a fairly constant hormone level so it may be that a continuous or extended cycle regime will be best in terms of irritable bowel problems. In other words you won't have a period for three months, or 12 months or at all. If you're already on a different type of pill, consider switching. If you're not on the pill then it might be a good idea to try the pill, and this type in particular.

If your irritable bowel symptoms began when you went on the pill, and if you can't find a brand that suits you better, then you seriously need to look at other contraceptive options. Vasectomy, female sterilization, the IUD, and the male condom used correctly, are all about as reliable as the pill and don't involve taking hormones. There's more on all of this in Step 7.

Living with an irritable bowel

Hopefully, some of the above will make a significant difference to your life. But it's probable that you'll be needing all of the Seven Step Programme and while you're working your way through it you still have to live with your irritable bowel. Here are some ideas to help you.

GENERAL TIPS

▶ Keep a diary in which you record what you eat and drink, your emotional state, and what irritable bowel symptoms you have. This may help you to identify the things that exacerbate your symptoms.

▶ Join an IBS support group.

▶ Contemplate the worst case scenario and plan for it, but remain optimistic.

- Experiment with the size and frequency of your meals. When you eat large meals, stomach distension triggers the gastrocolic reflex, causing your colon to contract. If you suffer from constipation large meals may therefore help. But if you suffer from diarrhoea it may be that smaller, more frequent meals (say five a day) won't be enough to trigger any bowel movement.

- Simethicone reduces the fullness, bloating and pain associated with intestinal gas. Tablets are normally taken four times a day after meals and at bedtime. Simethicone is sold under a variety of brand names. It's an anti-foaming agent which causes small gas bubbles to combine into large bubbles. It doesn't reduce the amount of gas but encourages it to pass out in fewer episodes.

- If your flatulence is embarrassing try cutting out all animal products because they're responsible for most of the odour (see Step 4).

- If you have IBS-D try not to give in to the urge to defecate until you absolutely have to. The longer you can hold on the longer your large intestine has to remove liquid and to normalize your stools.

- Explain your situation to family, friends and colleagues.

SCHOOL

- Discuss your situation with the school counsellor, who should make sure all the teachers know about your condition.

- In the USA you should consider a '504' – that's to say a plan drawn up under Section 504 of the Rehabilitation Act 1973. A member of staff will be responsible for '504s' and can work with you to make sure you're not disadvantaged by your condition.

- Confide in your close friends and enlist their support.

OUT AND ABOUT

- If you have IBS-D find out where all the suitable toilets are along the routes you have to travel – public conveniences, stations, cafés, restaurants, hotels and so on. Make your own 'good loo guide' so you always know where to go in an emergency.

▶ You may not be aware that there are 9,000 locked public toilets throughout the UK, exclusively for the use of the disabled. All can be opened by the same key and if you have severe IBS-D or IBS-M then you should qualify for one. Keys can be obtained for a small fee from the disability rights organization Radar, which publishes the National Key Scheme Guide, a handbook giving the locations of the toilets. There's also an app giving the same information. Contact information for Radar is given in the Taking it further section at the end of the book.

▶ In the USA, regulations regarding restrooms vary in different parts of the country. In some places it's accepted that even if you're not a guest you can use the restrooms in restaurants, airports, shopping malls, stores and hotels. In other places, even customers may be denied the use of a toilet in certain stores. The American Restroom Association has begun a Public Restroom Initiative (PRI) to make toilets more widely available.

▶ When you find a toilet there may already be people waiting. In the UK, the IBS Network as well as the Bladder and Bowel Foundation (see the Taking it further section for details) can provide you with a 'Can't Wait' card, which may help you jump a queue for toilets. In the USA, you may find it useful to subscribe to MedicAlert® and to carry the card as proof of your medical condition.

TRAVELLING

▶ Be very careful about what you eat the day before – keep well away from trigger foods.

▶ Get all your packing and paperwork done in good time so you're not stressed.

If you have IBS-D:

▶ Take Loperamide (Imodium™) before leaving.

▶ Get up early so you have time to empty your bowels before setting off.

- Prepare yourself an emergency travel pack containing Loperamide, soft toilet tissue, wet wipes, and a change of underwear.

- Consider wearing protective underwear.

- If your irritable bowel is exacerbated by travel sickness try ginger (see above).

YOUR ROMANTIC AND SEX LIFE

When you have an irritable bowel you're bound to feel anxious about relationships and sex. But you don't want to turn one problem (IBS) into two problems (IBS and the end of relationships).

- Dining out is a standard part of the dating ritual but it's probably something you'd rather miss. Come up with some other ideas – there's no need to be conventional.

- If you do eat out, or perhaps with your date's family, don't be afraid to specify the things you can't eat. Huge numbers of people nowadays restrict their diets for all kinds of reasons, including allergies, diabetes, religious beliefs and veganism. It's not something unusual.

- Avoid all animal products because they give gas its unpleasant odour.

- If you use a dating site consider including your condition in your profile so you only get replies from people who are relaxed about it. There is a dating site especially for sufferers: www.datingwithibs.com

- If you've begun a relationship with someone who doesn't know about your condition you'll have to decide when you're going to explain about it. That partly depends how severe it is and how difficult it is to hide it. Whatever the timing, don't make a huge issue out of it. The more you treat it as significant, the more your date will treat it the same way.

- When a serious relationship develops, make sure your partner fully understands your condition and knows how to be supportive.

- Don't get stressed about sex – that will only make matters worse.

- Make the most of your good days.

- Take the on top position so you don't have weight on your abdomen.

- When you're feeling particularly vulnerable you could perform oral sex on your partner as an alternative to intercourse or, if you're a woman, invite him to use the space between your breasts as a substitute vagina.

Case study

'I met a man just over two years ago and we had a baby together who is now three months old. But we didn't live together and in two years we only spent half a dozen nights together because of my fears about my irritable bowel symptoms. He didn't know I have IBS. He just thought I was a bit strange. The symptoms are at their worst in the morning and ease off in the evening, so that's when we would meet up. Having the baby meant I couldn't go on like that. So I told him and he just sort of laughed. I think he was relieved I wasn't hiding something even worse. We're now living together and it's going better than I ever dared hope. He brings me a hot water bottle when I have tummy troubles, makes me a soothing drink, and gives me a cuddle.' Cheryl (23)

Focus points

1 On your high street today you can buy various herbs, spices, minerals, probiotics, enzyme supplements, over-the-counter medicines and hormones (women only) that can make a significant difference to your symptoms.
2 Squatting to go to the toilet (rather than sitting) may tackle SIBO and several other conditions.
3 There are various gut irritants you should give up experimentally – you can always resume them if you notice no difference.
4 Start relaxation exercises and physical exercise right away.
5 Careful planning makes an irritable bowel easier to live with.

Next step

In this chapter we've looked at things you can do today at home to reduce your irritable bowel symptoms. In the next chapter we'll be looking at the things your doctor can do for you.

3

Step 3: Decide what you and your doctor are going to do

In this chapter you will learn:

▶ *How to deal with your doctor*
▶ *The tests that can pinpoint the cause of your symptoms*
▶ *What medicaments may help you.*

Doctors vary enormously in their attitudes to irritable bowel symptoms. At one extreme are those who believe it's 'all in the mind' and who secretly believe you should 'pull yourself together'. At the opposite extreme are those who fully understand how serious irritable bowel problems can be and who will try every possible treatment on your behalf. If your doctor is in the first category then, obviously, you need to move on to a specialist immediately.

More likely, your doctor occupies the middle ground. In that case you're going to have to be very persistent if you're going to get the best treatment. You'll help your case enormously if you read everything in this book and go to your medical appointments armed with as much information as possible.

Diagnostic test

So let's see what stage you've reached with the medical profession so far. Have you:

1   seen a doctor?

2   seen a gastroenterologist?

3   been tested for small intestinal bacterial overgrowth (SIBO) or been prescribed antibiotics for SIBO?

4   been tested for food allergy or been given a food challenge?

5   been prescribed antidiarrhoeals for IBS-D or any form of laxative for IBS-C?

6   been given a SeHCAT test for bile acid diarrhoea (BAD) or been prescribed medicine for BAD?

7   been tested for intestinal parasites or given medicine for them?

8   been tested for yeast (*Candida albicans*) in your digestive tract or given medicine to clear it up?

9   been prescribed antispasmodics?

10   been prescribed antidepressants or tranquillizers?

▶ If you answered 'yes' to all or most questions you've obviously been
  suffering irritable bowel symptoms a long time and received a
  good deal of expert medical attention. However, there may still be
  some useful ideas in this section for you.

▶ If you answered 'yes' to around half the questions you're well
  down the road of medical intervention but there are many
  options you haven't yet tried. Don't get frustrated or despondent.
  There are still treatments out there that could prove to be
  the solution.

▶ If you answered 'yes' to only a small number of questions, or none
  at all, you're obviously right at the beginning of your journey
  to solve your irritable bowel problems. There are a bewildering
  number of things you could try. In order not to waste time you
  and your doctor need to be very methodical.

IBS tests

Your doctor may not consider that any tests are necessary.
The attitude often is that if 'the cap fits' then you have IBS.
This is especially so if you happen to be a young woman
(because young women have a higher prevalence of irritable
bowel symptoms than men). However, that's not a satisfactory
situation. IBS is not a diagnosis. It's just shorthand for a
group of symptoms. It tells you nothing about the cause of
the symptoms. That's one of the reasons you need tests. The
other reason for tests is to exclude conditions that have similar
symptoms. They are:

▶ Inflammatory bowel disease (IBD), a group of inflammatory
  conditions of the colon and small intestine, of which the
  main types are Crohn's disease and ulcerative colitis (see
  below). Some doctors see IBD as an extreme form of IBS,
  while others consider it as something completely different.

▶ Ulcerative colitis, a chronic inflammatory bowel disease
  (IBD) that causes ulcers in the innermost layers of the colon

and rectum. Symptoms include abdominal pain and bloody diarrhoea. An IBS-type diet low in dairy, fat and refined foods, and high in fruit and vegetables will help. Drugs can be used to control the problem. Surgery may eventually become necessary.

► Crohn's disease, a chronic inflammatory bowel disease (IBD) distinguished by the fact that it can occur anywhere in the intestines and go deeper into the tissues than ulcerative colitis. The main symptoms are abdominal pain, bloody or watery diarrhoea, fever and loss of appetite. The same kind of regime that's suitable for IBS will also help calm the symptoms of Crohn's disease, that's to say, a change of diet, relaxation and exercise. Drugs can be used to control the problem. Surgery may become necessary.

► Coeliac (or celiac) disease is an extreme intolerance of gluten (found principally in wheat, rye and barley) which causes damage to the small intestine. Symptoms include bloody, fatty or foul-smelling stools, bloating, abdominal pain, constipation or diarrhoea, nausea and vomiting. Coeliac disease is easily confused with IBS but can be distinguished by tests. Treatment is the lifelong strict avoidance of gluten.

► Diverticulitis is inflammation of pouches (diverticula) in the gut, usually the colon. Treatment may involve antibiotics and a bland, low-fibre diet to allow the gut to recover. Soluble fibre can then be increased very gradually.

► Bowel cancer. Often there are no symptoms in the early stages. Later symptoms may include abdominal discomfort or pain, gas, a feeling that the rectum didn't empty completely, and either constipation or diarrhoea or both alternately. Diagnosis may involve colonoscopy, X-rays and multiple computerized tomography (CT) images.

If all these tests are negative and your doctor doesn't want to organize further tests you could try to nudge things along by saying things like this:

► I'm wondering if I could have a yeast infection.

► Do you think I could have low stomach acid?

► Is it possible I could be suffering from bile acid diarrhoea?

Your doctor might riposte by asking, 'What makes you think that?' So do your homework by reading all through this book. Then you'll be able to make a persuasive case. The fact is, these kinds of questions can only be answered by making tests.

Try it now

Read through the tests and drug treatments described in the rest of this chapter. Identify the test and the medicament you think most appropriate in your case. Go to see your doctor and ask for that test and that treatment, explaining your reasons.

Case study

'My problems began with bloating and indigestion as a teenager. In my early twenties, after the birth of my first son, things got worse and, at the age of 26, while I was pregnant with my second son, they got worse again. That was when my doctor first used the term 'IBS'. I'd never heard of it before. My doctor sent me for various tests. All were fine. At the age of 30, on top of everything else, I began to feel light-headed after meals. My doctor was stumped by that one. More tests. All fine. But I was losing a lot of weight and was scared so I began researching on the internet. That's when I learned about gluten intolerance. I had every symptom. I told my doctor but he just smirked. So I began my own gluten-free diet and within a few days I had never felt better in my whole life. In my opinion, a lot of doctors need to catch up with nutrition.' Tabitha (32)

ANTIBODY TEST

An antibody test will confirm whether or not you have coeliac disease, an autoimmune disorder of the small intestine whose symptoms include abdominal discomfort and pain, constipation, diarrhoea and fatigue. If you have coeliac disease it means you have an immune reaction to eating gluten, a protein found in wheat, barley and rye. The test will not work if you're already on a gluten-free diet (see Step 4). An endoscopy (see below) with biopsy of the upper small intestine may be used for confirmation.

ERYTHROCYTE SEDIMENTATION RATE (ESR) AND C-REACTIVE PROTEIN (CRP)

Erythrocyte sedimentation rate (ESR) and C-reactive protein (CRP) are blood tests that can be used to detect inflammation (as in the case of inflammatory bowel disease, for example). Sometimes just one of the tests is used, sometimes both tests are used to improve accuracy.

ENDOSCOPY

An endoscope (or simply 'scope') consists of a tube containing light and optical systems that, inserted into the body via, for example, the mouth or anus, allows a physician to see exactly what's going on. It can't be used to detect IBS but it can confirm or rule out other conditions which might give rise to similar symptoms, including visible inflammation, ulcers and tumours. An endoscope can also be used to perform biopsies and remove polyps.

Procedures vary. You might be asleep and know nothing or you might only be tranquillized. For an examination of your oesophagus, stomach and duodenum you'll not be able to have anything to eat or drink for between four and eight hours. You'll lie on your left side and the tube, about the thickness of a small finger, will be passed down through your mouth. There's no interference with your breathing. For an examination of your anal canal, rectum, large intestine and the final part of your small intestine, you'll have to follow a particular diet starting 48 hours beforehand, take a special laxative, and have nothing to eat or drink in the 12 hours beforehand. The tube will be inserted via your anus.

Between these two main kinds of GI tract endoscopy a huge amount can be seen, including the key SIBO areas, but there are around 5 metres of small intestine which can't be viewed with this technology (see the SmartPill below).

The results of the visual part of the endoscopy can be given to you in the recovery room but for any biopsy you'll have to wait a few days for the laboratory to report.

FOOD ALLERGY TEST

Both food allergy and food intolerance can cause irritable bowel symptoms. Unfortunately there is no reliable test for a food intolerance other than the laborious 'food challenge' – that's to say, eliminating all suspect foods from your diet for up to two weeks and then reintroducing them one at a time. However, your doctor can order various tests for food allergies including the skin prick test (up to 25 allergens at a time) and the Radio AllergoSorbent Test (RAST) on a blood sample (up to 30 allergens at a time). If an allergy is confirmed, or if a food intolerance is uncovered by a food challenge, then the standard procedure is to avoid the problem food or foods. However, it would be better still to tackle the cause of the body's abnormal behaviour. It might be an enzyme deficiency (see Steps 2 and 4) or it might be a 'leaky gut' – that's to say, a damaged gut wall that allows toxins, microbes, undigested food and waste to get into your bloodstream thus triggering an allergic-type response. Although there's a lot of good science to back up the theory of the leaky gut it's generally ignored or downplayed by the mainstream medical profession. As a result you may be left to treat your own leaky gut (see Step 4).

FULL BLOOD COUNT

Malabsorption of nutrients in IBS may lead to anaemia. A full blood count (FBC) will see if you have it. However, anaemia also occurs with other digestive tract disorders.

LACTOSE TOLERANCE TEST

Lactose is a type of sugar found in milk and milk products. If you're lactose intolerant you'll have irritable bowel symptoms. The two main methods are:

▶ The lactose tolerance blood test – several blood samples will be taken before and after you drink a lactose solution.

▶ The hydrogen breath test – breath samples will be checked for hydrogen before and after drinking a lactose solution, with a high post-drink level indicating lactose intolerance.

In the eight hours preceding the test you won't be able to eat anything or to exercise strenuously.

RADIOLOGICAL TESTS

Computed tomography (CT), magnetic resonance imaging (MRI), and ultrasound scans can reveal a huge range of problems in the digestive tract as well as in the gallbladder, liver or pancreas. If, in addition to the standard irritable bowel symptoms of bloating and gas, you also have pain in the upper right area of the abdomen, fever, nausea and heartburn, then gallbladder disease should be suspected and can be confirmed by radiological methods.

SALIVA TEST (WOMEN ONLY)

If you've noticed changes in your irritable bowel symptoms that are linked to your periods then a saliva test could be very useful. Such changes suggest a hormonal cause which might be treated via contraceptive pills (either stopping them, starting them, or switching to a different kind). All you have to do is spit into a plastic container during the second half of your cycle. A laboratory will then be able to measure the levels of oestrogen, progesterone, testosterone and cortisol. Based on those levels a specialist can tell which birth control pill will best reduce your symptoms, or may recommend you use a different type of contraceptive. For more on this see Step 7.

SIBO BREATH TEST

As you learned in Step 1, small intestinal bacterial overgrowth (SIBO) can be a cause of irritable bowel symptoms. Normally, the small intestine contains only a tiny number of bacteria but in SIBO they proliferate, causing gas, heartburn and other problems. The bacteria can be cleared very rapidly by antibiotics (see below) as well as by special diets. However, even if you opt for antibiotics you'll still have to follow a special diet to keep the bacteria from returning. For details of the dietary approach see Step 4.

Bacteria produce hydrogen. People do not. So measuring hydrogen in the breath is the standard test for SIBO, because the gas produced by bacteria in the small intestine diffuses into the bloodstream, is transported to the lungs, and is then exhaled.

Prior to the test you'll first have to follow a special diet for a day or so, eliminating the kinds of foods the bacteria like, and then fast for 12 hours. The actual procedure will be spread over two or three hours. There are two kinds of tests:

▶ **The lactulose breath test.** Lactulose is a synthetic sugar that can be digested by bacteria but not by people. The lactulose test is good at reflecting bacteria in the final part of the small intestine, where the problem usually lies, but not at the beginning.

▶ **The glucose breath test.** Glucose is absorbed in the first metre of the small intestine and therefore won't reach any bacteria further along. That means the glucose test can only reflect bacterial overgrowth at the beginning of the small intestine, which is less common than at the far end.

In general, the lactulose breath test is preferred, but it might be necessary to do both.

Remember this

Book your breath test for early in the morning so you don't have to be awake very long without eating.

THE SMARTPILL

The SmartPill is not a treatment but a capsule about the size of a raspberry which, when swallowed, relays detailed information about the functioning of the gut, including the section of the small intestine that's beyond the reach of endoscopes. In fact, your doctor wouldn't prescribe it in the UK at the time of writing because it's a very expensive technology. The Princess Grace Hospital, London, was the first to offer it privately in Britain at a cost of £1,750.

STOMACH ACID TEST

Low stomach acid is common in older men and women and can cause irritable bowel symptoms. The most reliable test is the Heidelberg Stomach Acid Test which involves drinking a solution of sodium bicarbonate after fasting for eight to twelve hours. A sensor put down into your stomach then measures how quickly and fully stomach acidity returns. If low stomach acid is confirmed it can be treated with tablets.

Try it now

If you haven't yet done a home stomach acid test turn back to Step 2 and follow the instructions in that section. You'll also find additional information about stomach acid in Step 4.

STOOL TEST

Using the latest techniques a huge amount of information can be uncovered by stool analysis, including the balance of microbes in your gut, yeast infection, parasites, inflammation, food sensitivities, intestinal bleeding, and even the degree to which your bacteria are resistant to antibiotics and drugs. So this is a very important test. If your symptoms are shown to be entirely due to, say, intestinal worms or yeast, then you can be cured by drugs.

Remember this

Not all doctors are the same when it comes to IBS. Attitudes within the medical profession vary enormously. If you don't think your irritable bowel symptoms are being treated seriously enough you must change to a different doctor or ask to see a specialist.

IBS drugs

On the basis of a physical examination, your history, and any tests that have been ordered, your doctor will prescribe treatment. Very likely that will include one or more of the medicaments described below. Hopefully they will work very well for you. Many IBS medicaments will have significant potential side-effects, however. If you suffer any of them you'll need to balance the upside (reduced irritable bowel symptoms) against the downside (the side-effects). Only you can decide whether it's best to continue or to seek a different type of treatment (see Step 2 and Steps 4–7).

In the descriptions that follow there's only space to mention the most significant side-effects. Always read the accompanying leaflet carefully to make sure any medicine is suitable and safe for you.

ANTIBIOTICS

▶ Why would my doctor prescribe them?

In some sufferers, IBS may be partly or entirely due to an explosion of bacteria in the small intestine – a condition known as small intestinal bacterial overgrowth (SIBO). SIBO can be treated very successfully with antibiotics and, indeed, in the early 2000s there was tremendous euphoria over the implications for an IBS cure. However, antibiotics have not proven to be as widely successful as had been hoped.

Controversy centres on the interpretation of the lactulose breath test (see above). In a healthy person, hydrogen in the breath does not rise until 90 minutes have elapsed since eating carbohydrates. In other words it takes at least 90 minutes for the partly digested food to reach the bacteria in the large intestine. A much quicker rise in hydrogen was interpreted as meaning that the bacteria were much further along the gut, closer to the stomach. In other words, in the small intestine. Some scientists are now questioning this. They argue that the early increase in hydrogen does not indicate that the bacteria are closer to the stomach but that the partially digested food is getting further from the stomach more quickly and reaching the large intestine much sooner than it normally would. In other words, an irritable bowel is a problem of transit time. Food passes too rapidly through the system. And, indeed, we know this to be the case in irritable bowel sufferers who have diarrhoea. When food moves too quickly there's insufficient time for water absorption and the result is watery stools.

So who's right? Although some doctors are claiming a success rate of 90 per cent for clearing SIBO, and an equally impressive figure for the reduction of irritable bowel symptoms, quite a number of studies paint a far less impressive picture. In well-conducted research in 2011 (Pimentel M, Lembo A, Chey WD, *et al*) patients with mild to moderate non-constipating IBS were either put on the antibiotic rifaximin or a placebo for two weeks. In the four weeks following treatment, 40.7 per cent of the rifaximin group reported adequate relief, so rifaximin is certainly achieving something. However, 31.7 per cent of the placebo group also achieved adequate relief.

Another way of measuring the efficacy is the Number Needed to Treat (NNT). If you've forgotten about NNTs see the explanation below. In at least one study, rifaximin had an NNT of 11, making it one of the least effective treatments for IBS. But NNTs and percentages are, of course, averages. Some IBS sufferers will have a better result and some will experience a more disappointing result. The bottom line is that rifaximin does have an effect, and for some people a very significant effect.

Key idea

We first met the Number Needed to Treat (NNT) in Step 2. Just to remind you, the NNT is a measure used by doctors and scientists to work out how effective a treatment is. It's defined as the number of patients you need to treat to prevent one additional bad outcome. For example, an NNT of 5 for a medicament would mean that out of every five patients treated there would be one more who recovered than if none had been treated. The key point to bear in mind is that the higher the number the less effective the treatment and the lower the number the more effective the treatment. Note that different studies may arrive at different NNTs.

▶ How do I take them?

Rifaximin (brand name Xifaxan in the USA) is the first antibiotic choice for this as it's not absorbed and remains entirely within the gut. It will not, therefore, have an impact on bacteria in other parts of the body. The usual course is 10 or 14 days. For IBS-C rifaximin might be combined with neomycin or metronidazole.

▶ Are there any side-effects?

Rifaximin is considered fairly safe but possible side-effects include allergic reaction, headache, nausea, dizziness, fatigue, bloating, and diarrhoea or constipation. Note that even if rifaximin is completely successful it can't stop bacteria re-colonizing your small intestine, which could start in as little as two weeks after the end of treatment. Therefore, antibiotic treatment of SIBO must always be followed up with preventative dietary measures. This is an important subject and the dietary approach is fully dealt with in Step 4.

ANTICHOLINERGICS AND ANTISPASMODICS

▶ Why would my doctor prescribe them?

The anticholinergics and antispasmodics are a group of medicines that prevent spasms and the ensuing pain in the smooth muscles of the body, including the gut. Some reduce irritable bowel symptoms by blocking special receptors or docking sites on the smooth muscles along the walls of the gut. Signalling chemicals can no longer communicate with those receptors with the result that contractions are reduced. Relaxants, by contrast, work directly on the smooth muscles to prevent spasms.

Anticholinergics/antispasmodics work for some sufferers but not for others. If one kind doesn't work for you it may still be worth trying another.

▶ How do I take them?

Antispasmodics should only be taken when needed. However, if you have, say, a lunch meeting coming up you can take an antispasmodic about 45 minutes beforehand so as to avoid problems. An antocholinergic such as dicyclomine, by contrast, is usually taken four times a day, half an hour to an hour before eating.

▶ Are there any side-effects?

Possible side-effects vary with the specific drug but can include constipation, drowsiness, dizziness, confusion, agitation, hallucinations, impotence, blurred vision, dry mouth and difficulty urinating. Avoid these drugs if you are pregnant, trying to get pregnant or breastfeeding. Make your doctor aware of any other drugs you're taking in case of interactions. Also tell your doctor if you suffer from congestive heart failure, difficulty urinating, glaucoma, hypertension, the neuromuscular disease myasthenia gravis, oesophagitis, ulcerative colitis or prostate enlargement.

ANTIDEPRESSANTS

▶ Why would my doctor prescribe them?

It so happens that tricyclic antidepressants (TCAs) are particularly good at reducing irritable bowel symptoms in about 85 per cent of sufferers. They have been in use this way for more than 30 years and are well proven. The fact that your doctor prescribes TCAs does not mean that you're depressed or that your symptoms are 'all in the mind'. The mechanism of action for IBS is quite different to the way TCAs work on depression. Other kinds of antidepressants are not as effective for IBS (although they might be prescribed in psychiatric doses where IBS *is* accompanied by anxiety and depression).

▶ How do I take them?

Your doctor may decide to start TCAs at a low dose (such as 10 mg a day) and then build up until you experience a sustained improvement in your symptoms. Generally a dose of 25–125 mg a day works well, which is below the psychiatric range for antidepressant effect.

▶ Are there any side-effects?

TCAs can cause numerous side-effects including dry mouth, blurred vision, constipation, urinary retention, impaired memory, drowsiness, dizziness, muscle weakness, nausea, low blood pressure, increased heart rate and sexual dysfunction. They are better tolerated if the dose is increased gradually. If you experience unpleasant side-effects which don't go away you'll be in the unfortunate position of having to decide which is worse, the IBS or the side-effects.

ANTIDIARRHOEALS

▶ Why would my doctor prescribe them?

Your doctor might prescribe antidiarrhoeals if you're suffering from IBS-D but not IBS-C. The most common antidiarrhoeal is loperamide, an opioid drug sold under various brand names, including Imodium® and Lopex®. It works by decreasing the activity of the myenteric plexus (also known as Auerbach's plexus), the major nerve supply to the GI tract. As a result, food moves more slowly, the time for water to be absorbed is increased, and the stool becomes firmer.

▶ How do I take them?

Loperamide can be taken as needed. If you have an important engagement coming up you can also take it in advance as a prophylactic (preventive) measure. Avoid coffee, which is a bowel stimulant.

▶ Are there any side-effects?

Although loperamide is indicated for IBS-D it should not be taken when diarrhoea is acting to rid the body of toxins or of organisms such as *E. coli* 0157:H7 or salmonella (or illness will be prolonged). It's not recommended for children under two. Taken on its own, loperamide will not cross the blood-brain barrier or, if it does, will not stay in the brain. However, there are certain combinations of drugs and normally innocuous things including black pepper and quinine that can allow the opioid content to act on your brain. If you feel 'stoned' after taking loperamide consult a doctor and provide a full list of the other medicines you're taking.

Key idea

About 9 litres of liquid enter the small intestine every day. About 2 litres come from food and drink and the rest from gastrointestinal secretions. Most of that, however, is absorbed leaving just under a litre to pass into the large intestine. When everything is functioning normally the majority of that is also absorbed, leaving only about 100 ml (about half a teacup) to be excreted in the faeces. In diarrhoea, matter passes so rapidly through the gut that there's insufficient time for the liquid to be absorbed.

Try it now

If your irritable bowel symptoms include diarrhoea you don't have to wait for a doctor before trying loperamide. It's available over the counter (OTC) at chemists all over the world.

ANTIFUNGALS

▶ **Why would my doctor prescribe them?**

Large numbers of people have the fungus *Candida albicans* in their GI tracts. It sounds alarming but this yeast normally gives no problems. However, it can grow out of control for various reasons and when that happens it causes, among other things, the classic irritable bowel symptoms. If your doctor suspects *Candida albicans* and it's confirmed by tests then an antifungal is the standard treatment.

▶ **How do I take them?**

Antifungals for *Candida albicans* in the gut are usually taken orally but some may be injected.

▶ **Are there any side-effects?**

In general, antifungals work by inhibiting fungal cell processes. Unfortunately, human cells use many of the same enzymes and pathways and antifungals may therefore have significant side-effects. Only take antifungals under medical supervision and read the information leaflet very carefully. The natural antifungals found in certain foods are safer (see Step 4).

ANTIHISTAMINES

▶ **Why would my doctor prescribe them?**

Your intestines include the same mast cells that are also found in your skin, the lining of your nose, your mouth, your tongue and the airways in your lungs. These mast cells are filled with granules containing histamine, leukotriene and chemoattractants. When you're allergic to something, Immunoglobulin E (IgE) antibodies attach to the mast cells causing them to burst and release the granules (a process known as degranulation). The histamine and leukotrienes cause swelling. When this occurs in the nose or the skin it's pretty obvious. When it happens in the GI tract it's not. You'll feel ill but, because you can't see anything, an allergic response in your digestive tract is probably not something you'll think of. If, together with your stomach cramps, bloating, and diarrhoea and/or constipation, you also tend to get the following, an allergy seems probable:

- Swollen lips or tongue

- Sore throat

- Heartburn

- Skin rashes

- Difficulty breathing through your nose

- Vomiting

- Distended haemorrhoids.

Antihistamines should reduce those effects.

How do I take them?

Antihistamines are normally taken orally. As they can cause drowsiness they're best taken at bedtime, if possible.

Are there any side-effects?

In addition to drowsiness antihistamines can also cause dizziness, nausea, blurred vision and confusion. They should not be taken with grapefruit juice (which affects absorption), alcohol, antidepressants or sedatives, or by pregnant women, those suffering from chronic bronchitis, emphysema or glaucoma.

ANTIPARASITICS

Why would my doctor prescribe them?

Intestinal parasites can cause, among other things, abdominal pain, cramping, bloating, flatulence and diarrhoea. It's quite possible your irritable bowel symptoms are entirely due to parasites, in which case you can be cured by antiparasitic drugs. Other symptoms of infection may include nausea, coughing, fatigue, dizziness, headaches and confusion. The problem is very common in developing countries – experts estimate that at least a quarter of the world's population is infected with intestinal worms alone. But it's also surprisingly common in developed countries. Dr Marcelle Pick, who founded the Women To

Women Clinic in Yarmouth, Maine, in the USA, says that 40 per cent of the women who come to her with irritable bowel symptoms are infected with intestinal parasites. A stool test will reveal whether or not your irritable bowel symptoms are caused by them.

▶ How do I take them?

The lifecycles of the various intestinal parasites vary enormously. You may be able to eradicate yours with a single oral dose of an appropriate drug, with two doses a day for three days or, at the other extreme, you may need three courses of 28 days each.

▶ Are there any side-effects?

Side-effects vary according to the particular drug but may include headaches, nausea, dizziness and, in some cases, temporary hair loss.

CHOLESTYRAMINE

▶ Why would my doctor prescribe it?

Cholestyramine will cure the type of chronic diarrhoea known as Bile Acid Diarrhoea (BAD), a little known condition. Some doctors consider BAD to be an aspect of IBS-D, others consider it to be a totally separate condition, and some may not have heard of it at all. If you have an urgent need to go to the toilet up to ten times a day and pass watery stools but don't have the other irritable bowel symptoms then you should ask your doctor to consider BAD. There is a test known as SeHCAT. This subject is dealt with in more detail in Step 7.

▶ How do I take it?

You'll need to take cholestyramine every day for the rest of your life (normally four to eight grams once or twice daily with a maximum of 24 g, as your doctor prescribes).

▶ Are there any side-effects

The most common side-effect is constipation but there's also an increased risk of gallstones as well as elevated triglyceride levels (a risk factor in heart disease and stroke). Over the long term there is sometimes tooth discolouration and decay. The drug may not be suitable for patients with various medical conditions, including diabetes and kidney disease. Other medicines should be taken at least one hour beforehand or at least four hours afterwards.

ENZYMES

▶ Why would my doctor prescribe them?

We looked at over the counter (OTC) enzymes in Step 2. Your doctor can prescribe enzymes that are more powerful. In particular, if your problems are due to exocrine pancreatic insufficiency you can be prescribed pancrelipase, a digestive enzyme combination of lipase, protease and amylase. The main causes of pancreatic insufficiency are inflammation of the pancreas (the symptoms of which are abdominal pain, greasy stools and possibly some anal incontinence) and cystic fibrosis.

▶ How do I take them?

Pancrelipase is normally taken with every meal and snack. Tablets should be swallowed whole with a full glass of water.

▶ Are there any side-effects?

Take care not to inhale any powder as it may irritate the nose or throat. Possible side-effects include dizziness, headaches, stomach pain, gas, nausea, constipation or diarrhoea, swollen joints and allergic reactions such as skin rashes and swollen lips.

ISPAGHULA (PSYLLIUM)

▶ Why would my doctor prescribe it?

Ispaghula is a fibre supplement that seems to be especially beneficial to some IBS sufferers, making it easier for food to move along the digestive tract and softening the stools, thus reducing pain and preventing constipation.

▶ How do I take it?

Ispaghula husk comes as a powder or as effervescent granules. It should be stirred into a glass of water after a meal and drunk straight away. One study (Kumar A, Kumar N, Vij JC, Sarin SK, Anand BS) concluded that the optimum dose was 20 g a day, but your doctor may have reasons for prescribing a different dose. Don't take ispaghula at bedtime. Always drink plenty of liquid throughout the day.

▶ Are there any side-effects?

If you have a problem swallowing let your doctor know. Because ispaghula will increase the bulk of your stools you may initially experience more discomfort but this should go away in a few days as your body adjusts.

Remember this

Never tell your doctor you're taking a medicament as prescribed if you've been missing doses or have secretly given it up. That will only confuse your own treatment as well as the treatment of people who come after you.

LAXATIVES

▶ Why would my doctor prescribe them?

If you suffer from IBS-C your doctor may prescribe a laxative. There are various kinds. Stimulant laxatives, the most common, cause muscles in the bowel to contract and move the contents along faster. As a result, less liquid is absorbed by the body and the stools are softer (see the Key Idea above). Osmotic laxatives work by increasing water in the colon, lubricating the contents and softening the stool. There is a special laxative which, at the time of writing, is only indicated for IBS-C *in women*. Known as lubiprostone (brand name Amitiza), it causes the intestines to secrete fluid, thus lubricating the gut, easing the passage of food, and softening the stools. However, its mechanism is different to that of osmotic laxatives. In technical jargon it's a selective chloride channel-2 activator. Bowel movements may occur within 24 hours of taking lubiprostone, while bloating and pain should be significantly reduced within a week. Andrews Salts are another type of laxative which also draw water into the bowel and have a mild action.

▶ How do I take them?

Stimulant laxatives tend to be used for short-term problems while osmotic laxatives tend to be used for chronic constipation. Lubiprostone comes as a capsule and 8 mcg is usually taken morning and evening with food.

▶ Are there any side-effects?

There's controversy as to whether or not it's safe to use stimulant laxatives regularly on a long-term basis. Some doctors say it is safe, others say there's a risk of damage to nerve endings in the colon and that, eventually, stimulant laxatives will cease to work because you'll develop a tolerance.

Osmotic laxatives can cause bloating, diarrhoea and dehydration and, in rare cases, kidney or heart disease.

Lubiprostone should not be taken by children under 18. It should not be taken by pregnant women, because there have been no studies on them, and it would also be prudent for women who are breastfeeding to avoid it.

In general, ispaghula/psyllium (see above) or a change in diet (see Step 4) is preferred to these kinds of laxatives.

LINACLOTIDE

▶ Why would my doctor prescribe it?

In 2011, linaclotide became the first guanylate cyclase-C (GC-C) to be approved by the United States Food and Drug Administration (FDA) for the treatment of IBS-C, as well as chronic idiopathic constipation (idiopathic means the cause is not known). Linaclotide thus became the first, new pharmaceutical approach to IBS in six years. It's believed to bind to receptors in the gut, increasing intestinal fluid secretion, speeding transit and reducing pain. Does it work? In a randomized, placebo-controlled study of 2,800 patients, abdominal pain relief was reported during the first week, reaching the optimum effect during weeks six to nine. Maximum effect on constipation was seen during week two. In another study of 804 patients by the University of Michigan Health System linaclotide performed significantly better than placebo over 26 weeks.

▶ How do I take it?

The dose for IBS-C is 290 mcg thirty minutes before the first meal of the day.

▶ Are there any side-effects?

Linaclotide should not be taken by children under six and is not recommended for children aged 6 to 17. The most common side-effect is diarrhoea. Other possible side-effects include bloating, stomach pain, headache, black or bright red, tarry stools and skin rashes.

PROKINETIC DRUGS

▶ Why would my doctor prescribe them?

The underlying cause of SIBO (see antibiotics, above) is thought to be a weakness of the migrating motor complex (MMC) which would normally sweep everything out of the small intestine, including bacteria, during the night. Prokinetic drugs (that's to say, drugs that increase movement) boost the MMC, and thus help keep bacteria out. They include erythromycin which is an antibiotic but which has prokinetic side-effects, and naltrexone (more often used to treat alcohol dependence). Serotonin modulators (see below) are also a type of prokinetic drug.

▶ How do I take them?

Dosing is quite complicated and needs to be left to your doctor.

▶ Are there any side-effects?

Erythromycin may cause abdominal pain, diarrhoea, nausea, vomiting, heart arrhythmia and allergic reactions. It should not be taken by women who are pregnant or trying to get pregnant. Naltrexone is considered safe at the low doses used to promote gut movement but sometimes causes abdominal cramping and diarrhoea.

PSYLLIUM

See Ispaghula (above).

SEROTONIN MODULATORS

▶ Why would my doctor prescribe them?

Serotonin is a neurotransmitter that, in the brain, is associated with happiness but which, in the gut, regulates intestinal movement. Patients with diarrhoea have been found to have higher than normal levels of serotonin in their blood after a meal, while patients with constipation have been found to have lower than normal levels. So this seems to confirm that serotonin has a role to play in IBS, especially as about 95 per cent of the serotonin in the body is found in the gut.

▶ How do I take them?

Tackling IBS through serotonin has some way to go, especially in terms of safety. Tegaserod (brand name Zelnorm in the USA) is a medicine for women with IBS-C and works by increasing the amount of serotonin in the gut. Approved by the United States Food and Drug Administration (FDA) in 2002, Tegaserod was withdrawn in 2007 because of concerns about an increased risk of heart attack and stroke. At least one subsequent study found no increased risk but it is now only available in the USA in emergency situations. Alosetron (brand name Lotronex in the USA) is also for women but works in the opposite way. It blocks the action of serotonin in the gut, thus reducing cramping, urgency and diarrhoea. However, alosetron is also restricted and only some doctors can prescribe it, due to the possible drug interactions and to the complications that can arise if you have other medical conditions. Prucalopride has been approved for use in some European countries and Canada but, at the time of writing, is not approved by the US Food and Drug Administration. Discovered in 1980, cisapride is no longer available in many countries, and was removed from the US market in 2000, due to fears over heart arrhythmias.

▶ Are there any side-effects?

Yes, potentially quite a few, so these are medicaments you would probably only use if other treatments have failed, and then only in close consultation with your doctor.

TRANQUILLIZERS

▶ Why would my doctor prescribe them?

Since irritable bowel symptoms are made worse by stress and anxiety, tranquillizers would seem to be an obvious treatment. However, they haven't worked very well in trials. Nevertheless it's possible that in specific cases doctors may have reasons for prescribing them.

▶ How do I take them?

Dosages vary widely. Your doctor will tell you what's appropriate in your case.

▶ Are there any side-effects?

Common side-effects include confusion, drowsiness, dizziness, faintness, weakness, blurred vision, slurred speech, skin rashes, constipation, allergic reactions and a loss of interest in sex. But other serious side-effects are possible.

Remember this

All drugs have side-effects but they quite often diminish as the body adjusts. Before you can decide whether to continue with a drug treatment or not you need to give it a fair trial. Only then can you compare the positive against the negative.

Focus points

1 If your doctor isn't interested in IBS find another doctor or see a specialist.
2 Be persistent with your health care provider – it can take time to discover the right medicaments for you.
3 Your doctor should carry out tests to eliminate conditions with similar symptoms.
4 But you'll also want tests to try to pinpoint the cause of your symptoms.
5 You'll need to weigh up the benefits of medicaments against the side-effects you experience.

Next step

This chapter has been all about the things your doctor can do for you. In the next chapter we'll be looking at one of the most important things you can do for yourself and that's modify your diet.

4

Step 4: Take control of your diet

In this chapter you will learn:

- ▶ *How certain foods cause irritable bowel symptoms*
- ▶ *Diets that can eliminate irritable bowel symptoms*
- ▶ *How to cure small intestinal bacterial overgrowth (SIBO)*
- ▶ *The truth about gas*
- ▶ *Why a leaky gut could be implicated in your problems.*

It seems pretty obvious that your irritable bowel symptoms have some sort of connection with the food you eat. For whatever reason, you can't tolerate some of the foods that other people eat without problems. So all you have to do is eliminate those foods from your diet and the symptoms will go away. Simple!

Unfortunately, it's not so simple in practice. Trying to identify the problem foods can be a long, frustrating, and, if it's not done right, ultimately pointless exercise. Getting at the truth isn't helped by the fact that a lot of 'politics' crops up whenever food is the subject of investigation. The processed food industry doesn't want to accept that its products could be in any way to blame. Vegans don't want to accept that too much insoluble fibre could be a problem. Lovers of fast food refuse to believe that fat could play a role. There's a lot of misinformation and poor science.

Attempts to discover which are the 'dangerous' foods has resulted in a bewildering dozen or so recognized IBS diets. The fact that they all have their supporters only goes to underline that IBS is not a specific disease but a range of disorders, each with its own treatment. Which is the one for you? You might come up with the right answer by luck but you're far more likely to be successful if you keep a detailed food diary. It can seem like a chore but it's a vital aid to you getting better.

There's a lot of information in this chapter and it can all seem to be very complicated. So at the end of the chapter I'll be looking for common elements in these diets to see if we can create a 'universal IBS diet' that will work for you and everyone. If you like you can skip to 'Making sense of it all' at the end of the chapter. But I strongly recommend you to read through the whole chapter because the better your understanding of the digestive process the greater the likelihood that you'll be able to uncover the nutritional regime that works best for you.

First, let's try to discover precisely what's going on in your particular case.

? Diagnostic test

1 I:

  a eat fast food several times a week.
  b eat fast food about once a week.
  c rarely eat fast food.

2 I:

  a eat fried foods most days.
  b eat fried foods a couple of times a week.
  c rarely eat fried foods.

3 I:

  a eat pretty much nothing but processed foods and prepared meals.
  b eat some processed foods or a prepared meal most days.
  c rarely eat processed foods or prepared meals.

4 I:

  a consume dairy products (milk, butter, cheese, eggs) most days.
  b consume dairy products a couple of times a week.
  c rarely consume dairy products.

5 I:

  a don't eat much soluble fibre*.
  b eat some foods containing soluble fibre every day.
  c eat plenty of soluble fibre.

(*Foods high in soluble fibre include good white bread, rice, soya, potatoes and bananas. For more on soluble fibre see below.)

6 I:

  a eat a lot of insoluble fibre*.
  b eat moderate amounts of insoluble fibre.
  c eat very little insoluble fibre.

(*Foods high in insoluble fibre generally include those that have a protective shell or which are tough or stringy such as nuts, seeds, whole grains and certain vegetables and fruits. For more on insoluble fibre see below.)

7 I:

   a consume a lot of caffeine every day (coffee, tea, colas, energy drinks and plain chocolate).

   b consume caffeine a few times a week.

   c consume very little caffeine.

8 I:

   a have a lot of fizzy drinks.

   b have no more than one fizzy drink a day.

   c rarely have fizzy drinks.

9 I:

   a believe I may have an allergy or intolerance as regards certain foods but I've no idea which ones.

   b have identified at least some foods to which I'm allergic or intolerant and avoid them as much as possible.

   c know I have no allergy or intolerance as regards any foods.

10 The food I eat:

   a is highly flavoured with lots of herbs, spices, garlic and onions.

   b includes herbs, spices, garlic and onions at least once or twice a week.

   c never contains herbs, spices, garlic or onions.

Your score:

You've probably guessed that 'a' answers are bad, 'b' answers are less than good and 'c' answers are broadly ideal (although what works for some people may not work for others). If you didn't score mostly 'c' then you need to read this chapter very carefully. You'll find an explanation for everything below.

The anti-inflammatory diet

It was long believed that inflammation played no role in IBS because colonoscopies and blood tests always came back negative. However, with more painstaking biopsies and microscopic studies it's now clear that low-grade inflammation does play a significant role (see Step 1).

Not just every IBS sufferer but every person should follow an anti-inflammatory diet. However, as someone with irritable bowel symptoms you may need to make certain adjustments to the standard anti-inflammatory formula, such as cutting out whole grains. Make an anti-inflammatory diet part of your lifestyle and then add to it one or more of the diets that follow.

To reduce inflammation cut down on:

▶ Alcohol

▶ Omega-6 fatty acids (in meat, margarine and many vegetable oils especially corn oil, safflower oil and sunflower oil)

▶ Trans-fats (in many processed foods, fast foods and commercial baked products)

▶ Refined carbohydrates (such as white bread and pasta)

▶ Fatty meat and red meat

▶ Full-fat dairy

▶ Sugar

▶ Food additives.

Increase your intake of:

▶ Omega-3 fatty acids (in oily fish such as anchovies, herring, mackerel, salmon and sardines, as well as in flaxseed oil and walnut oil)

▶ Fruit especially berries (cranberries, blackberries, blueberries, raspberries and strawberries), pineapple and papaya

▶ Vegetables (especially broccoli, cauliflower, sweet potatoes and spinach*)

▶ Whole grains*

▶ Ginger

▶ Organic sea vegetables containing fucoidan (such as arame, kombu, limu moui and wakame)

- Enoki, maitake, oyster and shiitake mushrooms

- Extra virgin olive oil

- Green tea

- Turmeric

* Note that whole grains cause problems for some irritable bowel sufferers (see non-grain diets below) and that spinach causes diarrhoea in susceptible individuals.

The low-fat diet

The low-fat diet is the simplest to implement. For many people, and especially for irritable bowel sufferers, fat has a very particular effect, as sketched out above. As soon as fat hits the stomach or duodenum (the beginning of the small intestine, immediately next to the stomach) it triggers contractions in the whole digestive tract, and particularly the sigmoid colon (the final part of the large intestine). If you're particularly sensitive to those contractions, as many irritable bowel sufferers are, you'll feel discomfort and even pain. If the contractions are uncoordinated (again, as is often the case with an irritable bowel) you'll experience bloating, cramps and, possibly, severe pain.

Why does it happen? Basically, the 'brain' in your digestive tract is readying your gut for action and moving waste towards the rectum so it can be eliminated to make room for the new meal. In some people either those contractions are excessive or, due to hypersensitivity, they're felt to be excessive.

Fat is not always apparent. According to Professor Eugene Chang from the University of Chicago, milk fat is especially prevalent in processed foods and confectionery, and poses a particular problem because it alters the composition of bacteria in the gut. The sulphur-rich bile that's required for the digestion of milk fat causes a gut microbe called *Bilophila wadsworthia* to bloom, he says, and leaky gut syndrome is the result (a condition in which microbes and toxins can get through the gut wall into the bloodstream – see below).

To follow the low-fat diet you need to give up or severely limit:

- Meat
- The dark flesh and the skin of poultry
- Dairy products (and processed foods containing them)
- Egg yolks
- Anything deep fried or battered, including chips, onion rings, fish and chicken legs
- All oils and fats
- Mayonnaise and salad dressings
- Solid chocolate and carob
- Nuts and nut butters
- Olives
- Coconut milk and fat
- Bakery products.

Key idea

It will help reduce fat if you:
- steam, boil or grill (without fat) rather than fry
- use non-stick pans to minimize the oil needed when frying.

▶ How do I know if I need a low-fat diet?

To find out if you have an exaggerated reaction to fat, test yourself on different kinds over a few days. On the first day, for example, swallow a couple of teaspoons of vegetable oil on an empty stomach and see what happens. The next day try lard. The next some high-fat cheese. If the reaction is violent you know you need to follow the low-fat diet to reduce symptoms. If you get no reaction then this is not the diet for you.

The low-carbohydrate diet

Here's something that may startle you. You're inhabited by more microorganisms than you have cells in your body. You have about 100 trillion in your large intestine and they'll be spread between 300 and 1,000 species, with 30 to 40 species dominating. Together they weigh about four pounds and, passed out alive or dead, they comprise about 60 per cent of the dry mass of your faeces. Whenever you feed these bacteria they proliferate and produce large quantities of gas. Of course, you don't deliberately feed them. But these bacteria love carbohydrates. Whenever you eat carbohydrates you're feeding the bacteria and adding to your gas problems.

The solution to at least one of your irritable bowel symptoms, then, seems very simple. Stop eating carbohydrates. In fact, not all carbs are equal when it comes to an irritable bowel. So let's try to understand a little more about them.

Basically, anything that isn't a protein (for example, meat) or a fat (for example, olive oil) is a carbohydrate. They come in three main kinds:

▶ **Simple carbohydrates** (abundant, for example, in fruit, vegetables, milk and anything made with white flour). They're digested in the small intestine of a 'normal' person and enter the bloodstream very quickly, causing a 'sugar spike' (which is not healthy).

▶ **Complex carbohydrates** (abundant in root vegetables and grains). They can also be digested in the small intestine of a 'normal' person, but more slowly, thus keeping the blood sugar level more stable (which is healthy).

▶ **Fibre** (abundant in vegetables, fruit and grains). Little changed in the small intestine, but provides food and a beneficial environment for bacteria in the large intestine. Gives almost no calories and therefore no energy.

Now the solution seems even clearer. If the bacteria live in the large intestine and need fibre to survive then all you have to do is cut right down on fibre which, after all, provides you with no energy anyway.

Unfortunately, it's not that simple. Your health is closely associated with the lives of those tiny creatures. They're not just along for the ride. They perform various useful and even vital functions such as:

- fermenting (digesting) food residue

- boosting the immune system

- preventing allergies

- creating vitamins (especially biotin and vitamin K), enzymes, neurotransmitters, amino acids and short-chain fatty acids

- nourishing the epithelial cells (the lining) of the large intestine. *Bifidobacteria* and *Lactobacillus plantarum* (abundant in fermented vegetables) are particularly good at this. If the walls of the large intestine are not properly nourished they become more permeable, letting toxins into the bloodstream and causing low-grade inflammation throughout the body.

- protecting you against food poisoning

- regulating your temperament (yes, they really do).

Although you lived without intestinal bacteria when you were in the womb, you probably couldn't survive without them now. So you can't kill them. But you could possibly reduce their numbers by starving them. That's where a low-fibre regime comes in.

The low- (and high-) fibre diet

What constitutes a low fibre regime? Nutritionists generally recommend around 21–25 g of fibre a day for women and 30–38 g a day for men. To give you an idea, a banana contains around 3 g of fibre, half a cup of peas contains around 4 g and half a cup of lentils contains around 5 g. So it's not that easy to get a lot of fibre. It may be that you're unwittingly already on a low-fibre diet. The average American or Briton, for example, only gets about 15 g a day.

There isn't just one kind of low-fibre diet because there isn't just one kind of fibre. There are two, soluble and insoluble. Here's the difference.

Soluble fibre:

► dissolves in water

► is completely or partially fermented in the large intestine by the action of bacteria, which produce gas (the more soluble fibre, the more bacteria and the more gas)

► slows the passage of food through the gut

► reduces the likelihood of diarrhoea

► softens the stool and makes it easier to pass

► lowers 'bad' LDL cholesterol and total cholesterol.

Insoluble fibre:

► does not dissolve in water

► passes through the GI tract only a little changed and is not therefore responsible for much gas

► speeds the passage of food through the gut

► adds bulk to the stool (it can hold 15 times its own weight of water)

► gives the muscles of the gut a good workout

► may protect against bowel cancer

► reduces the risk of developing haemorrhoids

► can irritate the intestines

► increases the likelihood of diarrhoea.

How can you tell one type from the other? If a vegetable or fruit seems stringy or tough or incorporates a protective shell of some kind then expect it to be high in the insoluble type of fibre.

High insoluble-fibre foods include:

Apples with the skin	Broccoli
Apricots	Cauliflower
Aubergine (eggplant)	Celery

Corn	Nuts
Beans	Onions, garlic, shallots, leeks
Berries	Peaches and nectarines
Cherries	Peas
Citrus fruits	Peppers
Cucumbers	Pineapple
Dates	Prunes
Grapes	Raisins
Green beans	Rhubarb
Greens of all sorts	Seeds and sprouted seeds
Herbs (fresh)	Tomatoes
Lentils	Whole grains
Melons	Wholewheat flour
Muesli	Wholewheat bread or cereal

High soluble-fibre foods include:

Applesauce	Mushrooms
Avocados	Oatmeal
Bananas	Papayas
Barley	Pasta/noodles
Beets	Potatoes
Bread (white and not industrial)	Quinoa
	Rice and rice cereals
Carrots	Parsnips
Chestnuts	
Corn meal	Soya
	Squash and pumpkins
Mangoes	

Swede (rutabaga in North America)	Tortillas made from flour
Sweet potatoes	Turnips
	Yams

Key idea

You can reduce the insoluble fibre content of fruit and vegetables by peeling them. Some people find it best to eat high soluble fibre foods first and high insoluble fibre foods last – so salad should come half way through a meal and fruit salad should come at the end. (The French typically serve green salad between courses.)

Case study

'I'd always been very health conscious and, for example, always insisted on wholemeal bread. When I began developing IBS I noticed that bread caused my IBS to flare up and assumed it was something to do with the gluten. So I kept away from bread altogether. Then one day for some reason I can't remember I found myself eating a slice of white toast and ... nothing. No IBS pains. So another day I tried more white bread. Still nothing. I discovered the problem wasn't the gluten but the insoluble fibre. Nowadays I cut right down on insoluble fibre and it's very rare that I get IBS pain.' Debbie (22)

▶ **How do I know if I need a low-fibre diet – and which one?**

Many irritable bowel sufferers have found that cutting back on fibre helps them. In a healthy intestine the two types of fibre work together to provide the ideal transit time, with soluble fibre slowing the passage of food and insoluble fibre speeding it up. But your intestine is not healthy:

▶ if your problems include diarrhoea but not gas; then it may be okay to continue with soluble fibre but cut right down on insoluble fibre.

▶ if your problems are constipation and gas; then it may be okay to continue with insoluble fibre but cut right down on soluble fibre.

However, there are various problems with a low-fibre regime. When you cut back on fibre which, as we've seen, contributes almost no calories, you're bound to eat more of foods that do contain calories. Removing that apple from your menu, for example, immediately reduces your fibre intake by around 3g, but your energy intake by only around 60 calories. Replace the apple with a croissant and jam and you've increased your net energy intake by around 200 calories. So cutting out fibre isn't helpful to weightwatchers.

The second point is that friendly bacteria do all the good things for you described above. If you only have the average fibre intake of around 15 g a day or less (that is, you don't eat a lot of vegetables, whole grains or fruit) you may well benefit from increasing it. That's something that must be done gradually, to allow your body and your bacteria time to adjust.

That brings us to the third and perhaps most important point. Your problem may not be entirely in the large intestine. It may also be in the small intestine where the walls can also become more permeable or 'leaky'. Normally there shouldn't be many bacteria in your small intestine but when you have an irritable bowel there are sometimes a lot, a condition known as small intestinal bacterial overgrowth (SIBO). Those bacteria in the small intestine feed not on fibre but on simple and complex carbohydrates – and that calls for a more sophisticated kind of low-carbohydrate approach.

SIBO

In a healthy person, the large intestine contains around a trillion bacteria per millilitre of fluid while the small intestine contains only ten thousand per millilitre – that's only one hundred thousandth as many. The healthy small intestine is virtually sterile. What's more, in a healthy gut, the profile of the bacteria in the small intestine is different to the profile of the bacteria in the large intestine. In the case of small intestinal bacterial overgrowth (SIBO), the number in the small intestine rises to one hundred thousand per millilitre or more, that's at least ten times normal, and they're the same kinds of bacteria as found in the large intestine. In other words, there are too many of the wrong bacteria in the wrong place.

Why would that matter? SIBO can lead to:

▶ **Gas in the small intestine.** Bacteria produce gas and the more bacteria the more gas, but the small intestine isn't designed to handle it in the way that the colon is.

▶ **Leaky gut.** This means that partially-digested food particles, toxins and the bacteria themselves can pass into the bloodstream causing allergies, chronic fatigue and pain.

▶ **Anaemia.** This is because the bacteria in the small intestine consume the iron and vitamin B12 in your food.

▶ **Fatty stools and deficiency of vitamins A and D.** This is because the bacteria decrease fat absorption.

▶ **Neurological damage.** This is due to the acids the bacteria produce.

▶ **Constipation.** This is because the methane gas produced by the bacteria slows the digestive tract.

So how do these bacteria get into the wrong place? There are several possibilities.

▶ When the small intestine is more or less empty, muscular waves normally pass along it to sweep bacteria out, together with any remaining matter. If you have an irritable bowel it seems these waves, known as the migrating motor complex (MMC), are too weak to do the job properly. Prokinetic drugs and serotonin modulators can help (see Step 3).

▶ Stomach acid may be too weak to kill bacteria on food. As we've seen, the strength of stomach acid decreases with age and also with the use of anti-ulcer/heartburn medicines such as proton pump inhibitors (PPIs) and histamine type 2 receptor blockers (H2RAs). So getting off PPIs and H2RAs would be a good idea, if possible. To increase the strength of your stomach acid take apple cider vinegar (ACV) or Betane HCL tablets (see Step 2).

▶ There's a valve between the large and small intestines, known as the ileocecal (IC), which is supposed to stop them. But the valve can leak. One possible cause of that leaking is straining while defecating which has the effect of forcing waste matter backwards from the large intestine against the valve. Always try to relax when you go to the toilet – squatting may help, as described in Step 2. There's also an ileocecal massage technique you can try and it's described below.

Try it now

To locate your ileocecal valve, imagine a straight line running from your navel to your right hip bone. The valve is roughly 7.5 cm below the middle of that line. Spend a couple of minutes a day massaging the area with circular movements of your fingertips.

Remember this

Migrating motor complexes are waves of muscular contractions that sweep through the intestines, flushing out indigestible particles as well as bacteria. They begin in the stomach after the digestion of a meal, at intervals of five to ten minutes, and each wave lasts for approximately one minute. If something is wrong with the MMC, bacteria in the colon may migrate back into the small intestine, causing SIBO. In order for the MMC to do its work don't eat between meals, late at night, or during the night, and postpone breakfast until you've been up and about for a while.

► How do I know if I need a SIBO diet?

You should be tested for SIBO if you have either a doctor's diagnosis of IBS, or a self-diagnosis based on the test in Step 1, plus at least one of the following:

- ► Frequent heartburn or gastroesophageal reflux disease (GERD)

- ► Food sensitivities or allergies

- ► Headaches, fatigue and painful joints

- ► Fatty stools

- ► Restless leg syndrome

- ► Rheumatoid arthritis

- Fibromyalgia

- Anaemia

- Diabetes.

The SIBO test is simple and painless and can be arranged by your doctor. Turn to Step 3 for details.

It's also possible to see what's going on in the small intestine using a miniature camera. If it's put down the throat (endoscopy) it can reach the first part of the small intestine, while a camera introduced through the rectum (colonoscopy) can reach as far as the last part of the small intestine. So the key SIBO areas can be seen, although there are around 5 metres which can't be viewed.

If your SIBO test is positive there are three possible approaches:

1 Special antibiotics which will get rid of the bacteria in a few days (see Step 3).

2 The elemental diet which will get rid of the bacteria in two to three weeks (see below).

3 The SCD™, GAPS™ or FODMAPS™ diets which will gradually eliminate the bacteria over two years or more (see below).

CRITICISM OF THE SIBO THEORY

Dr Mark Pimentel, Director of the Gastrointestinal Motility Program at Cedars-Sinai Medical Center, California, has probably done more than anyone else to promote the SIBO theory of IBS. In one of his studies he found SIBO was present in 84 per cent of IBS cases. It seemed to be an open and shut case for four-fifths of IBS sufferers. Cure SIBO and you cure IBS.

But more recently considerable doubt has been cast on the incidence of SIBO. The controversy centres on the accuracy of the lactulose breath test. If a healthy person eats carbohydrates it will take a known amount of time for hydrogen in the breath to rise (because the food has reached the hydrogen-producing bacteria). A much quicker rise in hydrogen is interpreted as meaning that the bacteria are closer to the stomach than they should be. In other words, in the small intestine.

Other scientists now argue that the early increase in hydrogen does not indicate that the bacteria are closer to the stomach, but that the partially digested food is getting further from the stomach more quickly and reaching the bacteria in the large intestine much sooner than it normally would. In other words, a positive lactulose breath test is not reflecting SIBO but rapid transit. Food passes too quickly through the system. And, indeed, we know this to be the case in IBS sufferers who have diarrhoea. When food moves too fast there's insufficient time for water absorption and the result is watery stools.

So who's right? Although some doctors are claiming a success rate of 90 per cent for clearing SIBO with antibiotics and diet, and an equally impressive figure for the reduction of irritable bowel symptoms, quite a number of studies paint a far less impressive picture. Indeed, research conducted by Dr Pimentel himself in 2011 (Pimentel M, Lembo A, Chey WD, et al) found that patients with mild to moderate non-constipating IBS reported adequate relief from the antibiotic rifaximin in only 40.7 per cent of cases. That may sound quite impressive until you know that 31.7 per cent of those on a placebo also achieved adequate relief. So the case for SIBO is looking weaker than it did, or, at least, relevant to a smaller proportion of IBS sufferers.

Another way of measuring the efficacy of a procedure is the Number Needed To Treat (NNT). (If you've forgotten about NNTs see the previous chapter for an explanation.) In at least one study, rifaximin had an NNT of 11, making it one of the least effective treatments for an irritable bowel.

▶ So what should you do?

NNTs and percentages are, of course, averages. Some irritable bowel sufferers will have a better result and some will experience a more disappointing result. The bottom line is that rifaximin (the antibiotic that kills bacteria in the small intestine) does have an effect, and for some people a very significant effect, and therefore takes its place in the Seven Step Programme as a possible part of Step 3. But even if you do use it you've still got to stop the bacteria returning, and that's where SIBO diets come in.

The idea of SIBO diets is to feed you but starve the bacteria in the small intestine. Once they're gone you'll have to stop them returning, which means continuing with a special diet, possibly for the rest of your life.

Key idea

Don't think of being on a special diet as necessarily a big deal. In reality, we're all on special diets. You probably don't eat monkey or gazelle or deer, for example, but other people do. There are those who seldom or never eat fish. And there are people who go their whole lives without ever tasting an oyster.

THE ELEMENTAL DIET FOR SIBO

The first SIBO diet we're going to look at is the elemental diet because it achieves the most rapid results. But it's of the kind that pretty much kills bacteria throughout the entire digestive tract. An elemental diet is a commercial formulation in powder form that comprises amino acids (the building blocks of proteins), a high proportion of sugars, small amounts of fat, plus vitamins and minerals, and only needs to be mixed with water. It is, in effect, pre-digested and so rapidly absorbed into the bloodstream in the first half a meter of the small intestine that the bacteria don't get a chance to feed on it. It's essential that during treatment you don't eat anything else at all otherwise the bacteria won't starve and die. Once the small intestine is clear you will then go onto a restricted but more normal diet. An elemental diet is therefore only a short-term measure.

In one study at the Cedars-Sinai Medical Center in California, 93 IBS sufferers with abnormal lactulose breath test (LBT) readings were put on an elemental diet called Vivonex Plus. After 15 days the LBT reading was normal for 80 per cent of the patients and at 21 days the figure was 85 per cent, possibly indicating that the bacteria had been cleared from the small intestine. Those with normalized LBTs enjoyed a substantial improvement in bowel symptoms and even those whose LBTs did not normalize enjoyed some improvement.

▶ How do I know if I need the elemental diet?

If you tested positive for SIBO and your symptoms are severe then you need the elemental diet. If your symptoms aren't too severe you may prefer a gentler diet because:

▶ they taste horrible

▶ you can't eat any normal food for two to three weeks

▶ the high sugar content can cause problems for diabetics

▶ elemental diets can stress the liver

▶ your calorie intake will be very low, which could cause a problem if you're underweight

▶ elemental diets are several times more expensive than the food you would have eaten

▶ as well as clearing bacteria from the small intestine elemental diets also kill good bacteria in the large intestine.

Remember this

You may be puzzled that a product high in sugar (a carbohydrate) is being used to kill bacteria that feed on carbohydrates. The point to remember is that the sugar is in a form so rapidly assimilated into the bloodstream that the bacteria have no time to eat it.

Case study

'After six years of IBS I was diagnosed with SIBO and put on an elemental diet for 15 days. The stuff tastes awful and for the first few days I had terrible bloating and gurgling which made it difficult to sleep. I couldn't understand it. I was only having this liquid food and yet I was bloated. Someone told me it could be to do with the bacteria dying. Anyway, I never gave up and at the end of 15 days I was on cloud nine because it worked. I felt normal. It was marvellous. I just ate everything I could and was loving it. But two months later the SIBO was back and I had to do the elemental diet all over again, which was tough. Now I'm very careful about what I eat but at least my irritable bowel symptoms are much reduced.' Sophie (36)

SCD™ and GAPS™

Elaine Gottschall described herself as just an ordinary housewife until her four-year-old daughter Judy fell ill with ulcerative colitis, a form of inflammatory bowel disease (IBD) that can seem like a severe form of IBS. When the family doctor advised surgery to remove part of the large intestine Elaine began looking for an alternative. In New York she found 92-year-old Sidney V Haas M.D. who had developed a nutritional approach to intestinal healing. Within ten days Judy was showing signs of improvement and within months she was growing normally. So at the age of 47, Elaine decided to study intestinal problems and gained degrees in biology, nutritional biochemistry and cellular biology. Subsequently she developed Dr Haas's method and called it the Specific Carbohydrate Diet (SCD)™ (published as *Break the Vicious Cycle*, Kirkton Pr Ltd, 1994).

Essentially, on the SCD you can't eat:

▶ Grains

▶ Starchy vegetables

▶ Beans other than haricot beans and fresh green beans

▶ Lactose

▶ Sweeteners other than honey, stevia (sparingly) and saccharine.

Like Elaine Gottschall, neurologist and neurosurgeon Dr Natasha Campbell-McBride had a child diagnosed with a serious condition, in this case autism. She noted that he improved significantly on the SCD and focused herself on making it even better. She called her nutritional programme the Gut and Psychology Syndrome Diet (GAPS™)

The word 'psychology' appears in the title because she was especially interested in the gut–brain connection (the subject of the next chapter) and its implications for not only autism but also dyslexia, schizophrenia, dyspraxia (which makes it hard to carry out smooth, co-ordinated movements), attention deficit disorder (ADD), attention deficit hyperactivity disorder (ADHD), and depression. But, again, many IBS sufferers benefit.

Essentially on the GAPS diet you can't have:

► Sugar

► Processed foods

► Anything with artificial colourings and preservatives

► Grains (rice, corn, rye, oats, wheat, buckwheat, quinoa, millet, couscous, spelt, semolina, tapioca)

► Potatoes

► Sweet potatoes

► Parsnips

► Yams

► Beans and pulses (except haricot beans and fresh green beans)

► Soya products

► Milk (but soured milk products are permitted)

► Alcohol (except the occasional glass of wine)

► Soft drinks

► Coffee and strong tea.

► How do I know if I need the GAPS diet?

GAPS has improved the lives of many IBS sufferers and it may work for you. Eliminating gluten is an important part of it for many. Certainly, a study at the Mayo Clinic has shown that cutting out grains (and therefore gluten) improves the symptoms of IBS-D sufferers, especially those who are HLA-DQ2/8 positive, a genotype that also predisposes to Type 1 diabetes. GAPS allows unlimited fruit, which is good for vegetarians and vegans, but many people have a problem with fruit. If you know you do then the FODMAPS™ diet (below) would be more suitable. On the other hand, GAPS is very restrictive on grains, beans and pulses, which is hard for vegetarians and vegans. On this score again the FODMAPS diet may be preferable. But, of course, it depends what works for you.

FODMAPS™

FODMAPS is an acronym standing for fermentable oligosaccharides, disaccharides, monosaccharides and polyols, a group of carbohydrates a research team at Monash University, Australia, believes are to blame for irritable bowel symptoms. It all sounds very complicated but they are only names. 'Fermentable' basically means they are digested by bacteria. So, under this regime, there's no problem with proteins or fats and you can eat as much meat as you like (as long as you're not also fat intolerant) as well as fish. But note that milk does contain carbohydrates.

FODMAPS may be bad for you for two reasons:

▶ Your body may not be able to digest and/or absorb them which means (a) more matter remains in your gut, and (b) more gas is produced – both factors leading to bloating.

▶ They're osmotically active, which means they attract water and therefore further increase bloating.

▶ Why can't your body handle FODMAPS?

Normally, these carbohydrates are broken down by hydrolysis in the small intestine into molecules of glucose, galactose and fructose which are then carried across the epithelium, the gut lining, by what are known as 'transporters'. One speculation is that in IBS sufferers there could be a problem with the transporters. For example, if there's a problem with the transporters called GLUT 2 and GLUT 5, the fructose can't be delivered into the bloodstream and ends up instead providing a feast for the bacteria in the small intestine and, subsequently, the large intestine, causing gas in both. But there are other factors at work, too.

The FODMAPS diet should be followed strictly for six to eight weeks. If it works – and it brings about a significant improvement in about three-quarters of IBS sufferers – foods can be reintroduced one at a time to see what can be tolerated.

The acronym 'FODMAPS' encourages the idea that all of them are bad for IBS sufferers. But that is unlikely to be the case. You may be okay with disaccharides for example, but not with monosaccharides. So the lists of FODMAPS below are broken down further to give you more flexibility. Remember that:

▶ oligosaccharides include fructans and galactans

▶ monosaccharides include fructose

▶ disaccharides include lactose.

FRUIT YOU SHOULD AVOID ON THE FODMAPS DIET

▶ **Fructans**

Custard apple

Persimmon (Sharon fruit)

Watermelon

▶ **Fructose***

Apple

Mango

Nashi pear

Tinned fruit in natural juice

Watermelon

* Fructose is found in most fruits but is tolerated when those fruits also contain an equivalent amount of glucose (which makes it more easily absorbed). It's fruits with excess fructose over glucose that need to be limited under the FODMAPS diet.

▶ **Polyols**

Apple	Blackberries
Apricot	Cherries
Avocado	Longon

Lychee

Nashi pear

Nectarine

Peach

Pear

Plum

Prune

Rambutan

Watermelon

VEGETABLES YOU SHOULD AVOID ON THE FODMAPS DIET

▶ **Fructans**

Artichokes (Globe and
    Jerusalem)

Asparagus

Aubergine (eggplant –
    but some people are
    fine with it)

Beetroot

Broccoli (but some people
    are fine with it)

Brussels Sprouts

Cabbage

Chicory

Dandelion

Fennel

Garlic

Leek

Okra

Onion (brown, white and
    Spanish, fresh, in powder
    or in processed foods)

Shallot

Spring onion (white section)

▶ **Galactans**

Baked beans

Chickpeas

Kidney beans

Lentils

Soya beans

▶ **Polyols**

Cauliflower

Green capsicum (the type
    known as the 'bell pepper')

Mushrooms

Sweetcorn

OTHER FOODS YOU SHOULD AVOID ON THE FODMAPS DIET

▶ **Fructans**

Inulin (a sweet-tasting soluble fibre found in chicory root and other vegetable roots and used as an additive in many products as well as a prebiotic)

Pistachios

Rye grains and products

Wheat grains and products

▶ **Fructose**

Corn syrup

Dried fruit

Fructose sweeteners

Fruisana® (a natural fruit sugar sweetener)

Fruit juice

Honey

▶ **Lactose**

Milk (from cows, goats and sheep), yoghurt, soft cheese, cream, ice-cream

▶ **Polyols**

Artificial sweeteners (isomalt, maltitol, mannitol, sorbitol, xylitol)

Sugar-free or low-carb sweets, mints, gums and dairy desserts

If you're a dedicated carnivore, a FODMAPS diet is no problem. But if you're a vegetarian or vegan it can seem quite daunting. So here, for those of you who don't eat meat, is a list of some things you *can* eat.

VEGETABLES YOU CAN EAT ON THE FODMAPS DIET

Alfalfa

Aubergine (also known as eggplant – may not be suitable for everyone)

Bamboo shoots

Bean sprouts

Beans (green)

Bok choy (Chinese cabbage)

Broccoli (may not be suitable for everyone)

Capsicum (except the 'bell pepper')

Carrot

Celery

Chives

Choy sum

Corn (raw corn may bother some people)

Cucumber

Endive

Ginger

Lettuce (may not be suitable for everyone)

Marrow

Olives

Parsnip

Parsley

Potato

Pumpkin

Silverbeet

Spring onion (green section only)

Spinach

Squash (may not be suitable for everyone)

Swede

Sweet potato

Taro

Tomato

Turnip

Yam

Zucchini (also known as courgette - may not be suitable for everyone)

FRESH FRUIT YOU CAN EAT ON THE FODMAPS DIET

The following can all be eaten in moderation:

Banana

Blueberries (organic)

Boysenberry (organic)

Cantaloupe

Cranberry (organic)

Durian

Grapes (organic)

Grapefruit

Honeydew melon	Paw paw
Kiwi	Pineapple
Lemon	Raspberry (organic)
Lime	Rhubarb
Mandarin	Star fruit
Orange	Strawberry (organic)
Passion fruit	Tangelo

DRIED FRUIT YOU CAN EAT ON THE FODMAPS DIET

Most IBS sufferers can eat the following in small quantities:

Banana chips	Paw paw
Cranberries (unsweetened)	Pineapple (unsweetened)
	Raisins (may not be suitable for everyone)
Currants	Sultanas

GRAINS AND GRAIN PRODUCTS YOU CAN EAT ON THE FODMAPS DIET

Amaranth	Oats (small quantities)
Barley (small quantities)	Quinoa
Buckwheat	Rice
Corn (may not be suitable for everyone)	Sorgum
	Tapioca
Millet	

MISCELLANEOUS FOOD AND DRINK YOU CAN HAVE ON THE FODMAPS DIET

Alcohol (small quantity only and preferably clear spirit)	Golden syrup
	Lactose-free milk, yoghurt and cheese
Barley bran	Maple syrup
Coffee	Meat (except processed)
Fish (fresh)	Molasses

Nuts and seeds in moderation (not cashews or pistachios)

Oat bran

Psyllium

Rice bran

Sugar (white, brown, raw and castor sugar in moderation)

Sweeteners (only nutrasweet, sucralose, aspartame, stevia, saccharine), tic tacs, minties and regular gum

Tea (including herbal teas)

Treacle

Water

Key idea

Fructose is more easily absorbed if it's accompanied by the same amount of glucose. It's as if glucose has a security pass to get through the epithelial cells and can bring fructose along as a guest. So when you're eating anything with a lot of fructose but very little glucose try adding extra glucose to the dish.

▶ How do I know if I need the FODMAPS diet?

Research shows that a low FODMAP diet helps with all functional gastrointestinal disorders (FGIDs), not just IBS. In one study, 77 per cent of patients showed a sustained improvement in gut symptoms. In another study, when IBS sufferers were deliberately given high amounts of fructose and fructans their symptoms were worse. Yet another study demonstrated that FODMAPS increase the amount of water and gas-producing fermentable residues in the large intestine. So there's an excellent chance that this diet will work for you. However, it certainly doesn't work for everybody and some sufferers say it made their symptoms worse.

Key idea

When you give up certain foods the tendency is to eat a lot more of something else. When you're starting the FODMAP diet make sure you continue to have a wide variety of foods.

REINTRODUCING FOODS

The FODMAPS diet is not a total ban, except during the first six to eight weeks. Once your symptoms have gone away you should reintroduce foods one at a time to see if you can tolerate them or not. Each reintroduced food should be tested for four days with a gradually increasing portion size. For example, you might have just half a dozen kidney beans the first day, a dozen the next day, and so on.

The IgG diet

Dr Peter Whorwell, the world-renowned specialist in gastroenterology, recommends IBS sufferers to eliminate foods that cause an elevation in their IgG antibodies, one of the classes of proteins that identify and neutralize foreign objects such as viruses and bacteria. A study at the University Hospital of South Manchester in which he took part (Atkinson W, Sheldon TA, Shaath N, Whorwell PJ) randomized 150 patients and asked them to follow either a sham diet or a diet excluding all the foods to which they had raised IgG antibodies. Those who followed the true diet meticulously had a 26 per cent greater reduction in symptom score compared with those on the sham diet. There's a growing body of evidence to suggest that eliminating IgG reactive foods will also relieve heartburn, fatigue, migraine and eczema as well as combat weight gain. The list of IgG reactive foods (that is, foods to eliminate from your diet) is:

Almond	Beans (kidney, lima, pinto, soy, string)
Amaranth flour	
Apple	Bean sprouts
Apricot	Beef
Artichoke	Beet
Aubergine	Blueberry
Avocado	Broccoli
Banana	Buckwheat
Barley	Cabbage (white)

Canteloupe

Carrot

Casein

Cashew

Cauliflower

Celery

Cheese (especially cheddar, cottage, mozzarella)

Cherry

Chicken

Chile pepper

Clams

Cocoa beans

Coconut

Cod

Coffee

Corn

Crab

Cranberry

Cucumber

Eggs (chickens' and ducks')

Flaxseed

Garlic

Grape (red)

Grapefruit

Halibut

Hazelnut (filbert)

Honey

Kamut

Lamb

Lemon

Lentil

Lettuce

Lobster

Milk (cows' and goats')

Millet

Mushroom

Oat

Olives (black)

Onion

Orange

Papaya

Pea

Peach

Peanut

Pear

Pecun

Pepper (green)

Pepper (black)

Pineapple

Pistachio

Plum

Pork

Potato

Pumpkin	Squash
Quinoa	Strawberry
Radish	Sugarcane
Raspberry	Sunflower
Red Snapper	Sweet Potato
Rice	Tomato
Rye	Tuna
Salmon	Turkey
Scallop	Walnut
Sesame	Watermelon
Shrimp	Wheat
Sole	Whey
Spelt	Yeast
Spinach	Yoghurt

You should also avoid:

Most herbs and spices	Cockroaches
Various grasses	Dogs
Various moulds	House dust/dust mites
Cats	

The anti-yeast diet

It's not unusual to have a yeast living inside your digestive tract. It's called *Candida albicans*. As with 'bad' bacteria you can tolerate it perfectly well as long as it's kept in check. But if the fungus proliferates, a condition known as gastrointestinal candidiasis (GIC), then, among other things, it causes the classic irritable bowel symptoms of abdominal pain, gas, bloating, and constipation and/or diarrhoea. In severe cases the fungus grows roots or hyphae which penetrate the wall of the digestive tract, leading to a 'leaky gut'.

The possible causes of GIC include:

- Overuse of antacids, antibiotics, NSAIDs, or steroids
- Overuse of sugar and sugary foods
- Chemotherapy
- Contraceptive pills
- Nutritional deficiency
- Pregnancy
- Stress
- Weak immune system.

There are drug treatments for GIC (see Step 3) but it can also be tackled through diet. Cut out:

Anything containing yeast	Grains
Alcohol	Honey
Baked goods	Mushrooms
Carbohydrates (refined)	Nuts butters
Cheese (aged or blue)	Peanuts
Chocolate	Pickles
Citric acid	Soy sauce
Dried fruit	Sugar and sugary foods
Fermented foods	Vinegar.

At the same time you should include the following antifungal foods in your meals:

- **Clove oil.** A 2009 study (Pinto *et al*) concluded that clove oil and eugenol (the active ingredient) 'have considerable antifungal activity against clinically relevant fungi'.
- **Coconut oil.** Contains the powerful antifungal caprylic acid.
- **Garlic.** A 1988 study by Mahmoud Ghannoum at Kuwait University concluded that 'the growth of C. albicans was found to be markedly inhibited' by fresh, uncooked, crushed garlic.

- **Oil of oregano.** A 2001 study at Georgetown University Medical Center concluded that oil of oregano at a concentration of 0.25 mg/ml 'was found to completely inhibit the growth of Candida albicans'.

- **Citrus seed extract.** A study published in the Journal of Orthomolecular Medicine in 1990 (Ionescu *et al*) found that 'oral administration ... resulted in a significant inhibition of *Candida*'. Citrus seed extract (usually grapefruit) can be bought in the form of liquid concentrate or tablets.

During the first week you may feel cravings for sweet things. Be strong and fight against them. At the end of four weeks review your symptoms. If they're no better this isn't the diet for you. On the other hand, if you've experienced a significant improvement, keep on with it.

Key idea

To prevent *Candida albicans* from adapting it's a good idea to use two or three natural antifungals at a time and to vary them from week to week.

How do I know if I need the anti-yeast diet?

If you have GIC the yeast will probably spread to other parts of the body where its presence will be clearer. In one study (Krause *et al*), a researcher known to be free of *Candida albicans* deliberately swallowed a large dose. Within three hours the scientists were able to culture the yeast from the volunteer's blood and urine, proving that yeast travels throughout the body. If you're a woman who frequently suffers from thrush that's a strong indication that you probably have GIC as well and it needs to be cleared up if the thrush treatment is to be successful.

The more of the following you suffer from the more likely it is that you have candidiasis:

- Allergies to certain foods

- Athlete's foot

- Bladder infections

- Depression

- Fatigue

- Headaches

- Heartburn

- Kidney infections

- Mental fogginess or confusion

- Mood swings

- Muscle and joint pain

- PMS

- Sinus infections

- Skin problems

- Thrush

- Urinary frequency or urgency

- Vaginitis

- White coating on your tongue.

If you suspect GIC there are home-test kits you can buy but the best course is to ask your doctor for a test.

The paleo diet

The paleo diet is based on the idea that our genes predispose us to dealing with the kinds of foods eaten in Palaeolithic times. That's to say, what was eaten by our ancestors two and a half to three million years ago. Its leading advocate is Loren Cordain, a professor in the Department of Health and Exercise Science at Colorado State University, but other people have produced their own slightly different versions of the diet.

Palaeolithic people, Professor Cordain believes, had a diet higher in protein, fibre, monounsaturated and Omega-3 fats, potassium, vitamins and minerals than we do, and lower in carbohydrates and sodium.

According to this thinking, all kinds of problems, including IBS are caused by consuming:

- Artificial colourings, flavourings and preservatives
- Processed foods
- Grains
- Legumes
- Potatoes
- Dairy products
- Vegetable and seed oils (except those listed below)
- Sugar
- Salt
- Alcohol.

On the paleo diet you're confined to:

- Fresh, grass-produced meat
- Poultry
- Fresh fish and seafood
- Eggs
- Seasonal tubers, fruits and vegetables as well as fermented vegetables
- Nuts and seeds
- Avocado, coconut, flaxseed, macadamia, olive and walnut oils
- Herbs, spices, vinegar
- Drinks: water, tea, and home-made bone broths (plus alcohol occasionally, as long as it's gluten-free*).

*Some authorities say grain-based alcohols contain gluten, others disagree.

▶ How do I know if I need the paleo diet?

There doesn't seem to be any scientific research specifically into the effect of the paleo diet on IBS but two aspects are well-known to help many IBS sufferers:

▶ eliminating grains

▶ eliminating lactose (dairy).

However, the paleo diet does allow and even encourage foods that frequently cause IBS problems, including those high in fibre and fructose. So although it may help some, following a 'Stone Age regime' is of limited relevance in IBS.

The low-gas diet

Gas and passing gas (farting) are facts of life. Everybody, including presidents, princesses and film stars, produces gas and emits it via the anus in between 8 and 20 episodes a day. The volume varies enormously between healthy individuals, as well as from day to day, but is generally within the range of half a litre to one and a half litres in 24 hours.

If you want to know what that amount of gas looks like, find a large, empty soft drink bottle and imagine it inside your abdomen. It's not surprising if your waistband feels tight now and then.

The gas naturally comes from the air we swallow (a tiny contribution because it's mostly expelled by burping), from gas that filters out of the bloodstream and into the digestive tract, from chemical reactions, and from the bacteria that live and feed in the digestive tract (mostly in the large intestine).

Not all of the gas is emitted via the anus. Some of it, especially the carbon dioxide, is absorbed into the bloodstream from where it passes into the lungs and is then exhaled. Some bacteria absorb the gas produced by other bacteria, especially the hydrogen, in turn producing methane and sulphur-containing gases.

▶ So what's different about IBS?

Research into the volume of gas produced by IBS sufferers is contradictory. Some studies have found the volume to be within the normal range while others have found it to be up to five times higher than normal. In all probability IBS sufferers differ widely in this because, as has been emphasized many times, IBS is not a single problem but an umbrella term for many conditions. In one experiment, eating baked beans increased gas by 12 times, while lactose can increase it eight times in lactose-intolerant people, and soluble fibre by four times.

Two things are clear. Firstly, anyone at the top of the normal range is producing three times more gas than someone at the bottom, and that's got to be uncomfortable. Even if as an IBS sufferer you're only producing a little above the normal range, say two litres, that is nevertheless four times more than some people. Secondly, it's now known that the way gas moves in IBS sufferers is different. Gas normally moves freely along the gut independent of solids and liquids, and faster when you're standing up. But experiments using radioactive isotopes have shown that in IBS sufferers gas pools in the small intestine, especially the first part.

In another experiment, IBS sufferers and controls had gas infused into their small intestines. The normal subjects tolerated the gas very well, even up to an abnormally high rate of around two litres per hour, but the IBS sufferers did not. It also seems that 'normal' people have a reflex contraction of the abdominal muscles in response to increased gas pressure, whereas in people with IBS this reflex doesn't work properly. Strengthening the abdominal muscles might help (see Step 6).

So IBS sufferers just can't handle gas, ending each day with a much bigger waistline than they had in the morning.

Whether you're especially sensitive to gas or not, reducing gas-producing foods is certain to make you feel more comfortable, both physically and psychologically. So restrict:

▶ Beans

▶ Lactose (if you're lactose intolerant)

▶ Soluble fibre

▶ Starchy foods such as corn, oats, potatoes and wheat.

QUANTITY VERSUS 'QUALITY'

Odour is a completely different issue to volume. Some 74 per cent of the volume of gas in the intestines comes from hydrogen, carbon dioxide and methane, all of which are produced there. Twenty-five per cent comes from nitrogen, a major component of the air, and from oxygen. Methane, contrary to popular opinion, has no odour, nor do those other gases. It's the remaining one per cent that gives farts their smell.

It's been surprisingly difficult to pin down the precise source of the odour but scientists are now convinced that the main culprits are hydrogen sulphide (H_2S), methyl mercaptan and dimethyl sulphide. Humans can smell hydrogen sulphide at concentrations as low as 0.005 to 0.3 parts in one million parts of air. So it takes very little.

Which foods are the biggest cause? Popular humour puts the blame on vegetarians and it's true that various vegetables, including asparagus, broccoli, Brussels sprouts, cabbage, cauliflower, garlic, leeks and onions, do contain sulphur.

But the real villain is meat and that was proven by Elizabeth Magee, Caroline Richardson, Róisín Hughes and John Cummings who published their findings in the American Journal of Clinical Nutrition. They recruited five healthy men and fed them a sequence of five different diets for ten days each, ranging from zero meat on a vegetarian diet up to 600 g of meat a day. Sulphide concentrations in the faeces were found to be only 0.22 mmol/kg on the vegetarian diet but as much as 3.38 mmol/kg on the high-meat diet – that's 15 times more.

As an IBS sufferer this leaves you with a dilemma. It's the action of bacteria on undigested food particles (mostly fibre) in the large intestine that's responsible for the volume of gas. But it's meat that causes the smell.

Try it now

By keeping a record of when your flatulence is at its worst and what you've been eating you should be able to identify the food culprits in your particular case. Different foods produce gas at different speeds but as a rough idea it takes about three hours with maximum volume being reached after five hours. After seven hours the gas should have been expelled. (That's why bloating is often at its maximum at bedtime and its minimum first thing in the morning.) So if you have a lot of discomfort at, say, six o'clock then the problem food is something you had for lunch.

The allergy and intolerance diet

If you suffer from hay fever, allergic skin rashes, or have dramatic reactions to bee stings you probably already know about mast cells. As part of the immune response, mast cells release histamine and other inflammatory chemicals in a process known as degranulation causing, for example, hay fever or skin rashes. But mast cells are also distributed throughout the digestive tract. Researchers (Barbara G *et al* as well as O'Sullivan M *et al*) have found that irritable bowel sufferers have abnormally large numbers of mast cells in their digestive tracts, especially in the first part of the large intestine.

By allowing blood vessels to 'leak' at the site of an injury, mast cells help antibodies to get into the damaged tissue to fight disease-causing organisms. Unfortunately, mast cells sometimes respond to substances that pose no threat at all. When this happens you have an allergy. And when it happens in the digestive tract, the same leakiness and the same swelling can cause discomfort, pain and the interruption of normal functioning. In addition, whenever the allergen is eaten, the gut tries to get rid of it, producing diarrhoea and cramping. This is one instance in which there is a physical difference between the IBS gut and the normal gut, because IBS sufferers have been found to have higher than usual numbers of mast cells in the colon and small intestine.

A food intolerance is slightly different to an allergy. Symptoms include stomach aches, bloating, acid reflux, nausea, diarrhoea, depression and fatigue. Whereas an allergy is an immune reaction involving an IgE antibody response, a food intolerance is a non-immune reaction. An allergy test (which depends on the IgE antibody) won't pick it up. Tracking it down, therefore, can be a slow and frustrating business. But if we have to, we will.

Remember this

Allergens can crop up in all kinds of foods, drinks and even medicaments where they're not expected. For example, lactose is a common filler in pills. It could be that you think you're allergic to a particular medicine when, in fact, you're really allergic to the lactose used as a filler. The lesson is: always read labels with great care.

So is IBS simply a food allergy or intolerance? Well, a true allergy is something quite specific and is treated differently to IBS. But, yes, IBS is a food intolerance. The very word 'allergy' makes that condition sound worse but, in fact, the symptoms of an intolerance can be more unpleasant. In either case the symptoms may include the classic IBS problems of abdominal cramps, pain, gas, nausea, diarrhoea and/or constipation.

The main differences between the two are:

► A true food allergy is associated with Immunoglobin E(IgE) antibodies against the food, while a food intolerance is not. Standard IgE tests can identify allergens but not foods to which you have an intolerance.

► Food allergy symptoms usually develop suddenly within a few minutes to two hours of eating the food, whereas the symptoms of a food intolerance come on gradually and may not be apparent for 24 hours or so.

► A food intolerance may cause neurological symptoms such as irritability, nervousness, aggression, dizziness, headaches and the feeling of not being in full control of your body. A food allergy does not.

If you have other symptoms in addition to your irritable bowel symptoms an allergy/intolerance should be suspected. Those additional symptoms might include skin rashes or swellings, breathing difficulties, raised heart rate/palpitations, and headaches/migraine.

If you have a true food allergy there's about a 90 per cent chance it will be due to one of the following:

Peanuts	Milk
Other nuts	Eggs
Fish	Soy
Shellfish	Wheat.

With a bit of luck and a food diary you may be able to track down the problem food. If it seems you have an allergy your doctor can arrange an IgE allergy test which may pinpoint the culprits. However, if it's a food intolerance the danger foods may be a lot harder to identify. The most common intolerance is to lactose. That's to say, your digestive system can't handle milk or milk products. However, it's quite likely you're not intolerant of just one or two specific foods but of chemicals that are in scores of foods. Salicylates and amines (see below) are likely culprits. What makes it hard to pin the problem chemicals down is that you'll probably be able to tolerate a certain amount of them and only get a reaction when the combined total from several foods reaches your threshold.

Given the difficulty of identifying problem foods, a better solution may be to come at the allergy/intolerance problem from a different angle. That's to say, rather than eliminate certain foods, stop the body reacting to them. There's an increasing amount of evidence that food allergy/intolerance is often caused by a leaky gut.

What happens with a leaky gut is this. The lining of the intestines has to be permeable to the right things otherwise you wouldn't be able to get any of the nourishment in your food into your bloodstream. A leaky gut allows some of the wrong things to make the crossing – bacteria, toxins and partially digested food particles, for example. As a result you can have all kinds of unpleasant and even dangerous reactions.

If you suspect you have a leaky gut there are tests that can confirm it. The standard one is to swallow the sugars lactulose and mannitol and measure them in the urine. Your doctor can arrange this.

So what causes the gut wall to leak? The problem is thought to be initiated most often by:

▶ Infection

▶ Overuse of alcohol

▶ Overuse of non-steroidal anti-inflammatory drugs (NSAIDs) such as ibuprofen or aspirin

▶ Overuse of antibiotics which kill friendly bacteria along with the bad

▶ Chronic stress (because it reduces the blood supply to the gut and slows repair of the intestinal lining).

Once the body has an allergic reaction to partially-digested food particles passing through the gut wall, so eating more of that food in turn increases gut permeability even further. It becomes a circular problem.

To heal a leaky gut:

▶ Give up alcohol.

▶ Stop taking NSAIDs if possible. If NSAIDs are essential, take nabumetone, the only one that, at the time of writing, does not increase intestinal permeability.

▶ Give up caffeine.

▶ Give up processed foods (which may contain harmful chemicals).

▶ Don't take antibiotics or eat meat from animals that have been fed antibiotics (that is, only eat meat from organic farms).

▶ Try berberine, a food supplement found in the roots, rhizomes, stems and bark of various plants, as an effective antimicrobial which can restore normal gut wall function. It has proven itself in the laboratory, in mice and anecdotally in humans although I'm not aware of any scientific studies using people.

▶ Take Betaine HCL (hydrochloric acid) to restore stomach acidity (see Step 2)

▶ As an alternative to Betaine HCL take apple cider vinegar (ACV – see Step 2).

SALICYLATE AND AMINE INTOLERANCE

Fruit and vegetables are widely believed to be healthy foods. And they are in many ways. But they also have their dark side. To protect themselves from attack, plants produce natural pesticides and some of them are quite potent. Many plants are high in organic compounds known as salicylates, for example, which protect them against fungi, bacteria and insects. The most famous salicylate is acetylsalicylic acid – better known as aspirin. Most people can handle a normal quantity of salicylates perfectly well but you may be one of those who can't. In fact, about 70 per cent of people with irritable bowel symptoms are sensitive to salicylates. In them they cause gastric irritation and diarrhoea as well as non-gut problems including skin rashes, swollen lips and tongue, wheezing and asthma.

Salicylates are especially found in:

▶ **Fruit**

Apples	Lychees
Apricots	Mandarins (A)
Avocados (A)	Nectarines
Blackberries	Oranges
Blackcurrants	Passionfruits (A)
Blueberries	Peaches
Boysenberries	Pineapples
Cherries	Plums
Cranberries	Pomegranates
Currants	Prunes
Dates (A)	Raisins
Grapes (A)	Raspberries
Grapefruits	Rockmelons
Guavas	Strawberries
Kiwis (A)	Sultanas

Tangelos

Tangerines

Watermelons

▶ **Vegetables**

Alfalfa sprouts

Artichokes

Aubergines (eggplants) (A)

Broad beans

Capsicums

Chicory

Chillies

Courgettes (zucchini)

Cucumbers

Gherkins

Olives (A)

Radishes

Tomatoes and especially
tomato products (A)

Water chestnuts

Watercress

▶ **Nuts and snacks**

All flavoured crisps and snacks (A)

Almonds

Muesli bars

▶ **Sweets**

Chewing gum

Fruit flavourings

Honey and honey
flavourings

Jam

Liquorice

Peppermints

▶ **Drinks**

Cordials

Fruit-flavoured drinks

Fruit juice (except pear)

Liqueurs

Peppermint tea

Port (A)

Rum (A)

Tea

Wine (A)

A = also high in amines
(see below)

▶ Miscellaneous

Fish and meat paste

Herbs and spices (with the exception of chives, garlic, parsley, salt, saffron, soy sauce and vanilla)

Vinegars except malt vinegar

If you're sensitive to salicylates it's very likely that you're also sensitive to amines. Amines are well known to cause headaches and migraines in sensitive people but they can also exacerbate irritable bowel symptoms. Certain foods naturally contain high levels of amines but because they're mostly produced by the breakdown of protein (amino acids), they can develop in all kinds of foodstuffs as they age.

Normally amines are oxidized by MAO enzymes in the gut (so anyone taking MAO inhibitors for depression must already be especially careful to avoid them).

The fact that you're sensitive to amines doesn't mean you can't eat any food that contains them. Everyone has a threshold. Most unaffected people can probably tolerate 100 mg whereas, in your case, it might be you can only tolerate 10 mg or as little as 5 mg. To give you an idea, the average banana contains around 1 mg but total amine content can vary enormously. For example, vermouth can contain as little as 0.25 mg/litre or as much as 9 mg/litre, while vinegar can vary between 1 mg/litre and 25 mg/litre (figures from the Nutrition and Food Science Unit at the University of Barcelona). You may have no problem with one kind of food or drink one day but a severe problem another day with a different batch or brand.

Amines are especially found in:

▶ Fruit

Bananas	Mandarins (S)
Figs	Pineapples (S)
Grapes	Plums (S)
Lemons	Raspberries (S)
Orange juice (S)	

▶ Vegetables

Aubergines (S)

Avocados

Mushrooms

Tomatoes and tomato juice (S)

Vegetable juice

▶ Drinks

Beer

Cola type drinks

Wine (S)

▶ Miscellaneous

Cheese (especially blue cheese but excepting soft cheese)

Chocolate (especially dark chocolate)

Dried, pickled or smoked fish

Offal

Preserved meats

Sauerkraut and fermented foods

Soy sauce

Vinegar (S)

Yeast extract.

S = also contains salicylates

Remember this

As food ripens or ages so the amine content can increase very sharply. Don't eat food that's stale, or has been stored for a long time, or that's over-ripe. Browning, grilling and charring food also increases the amine content – it's better to boil, steam or microwave.

Salicylate and amine intolerances are believed by some to go hand in hand with a third, which is glutamate intolerance.

Glutamate is an amino acid and excitatory neurotransmitter that occurs naturally in some foods including parmesan cheese, mushrooms and ripe tomatoes. As a food additive it not only improves flavour but also makes us crave more, which is why it's very popular with the processed and fast food industries.

The most famous additive is monosodium glutamate (MSG) but glutamate can appear under a number of guises including glutamic acid, umami and E621. In addition, the artificial sweetener aspartame converts to glutamate in the body. Although many people insist they suffer from 'Chinese Restaurant Syndrome' because of the amount of MSG used, various scientific studies have failed to find any harmful effects and the U.S. Food and Drug Administration (FDA) considers MSG safe in the usual quantities. So you can probably ignore this as a possible factor in IBS.

Try it now

There are two ways you can carry out food tests at home. Neither is perfect but they may pinpoint the source of your problems.

The first and simplest method is to rub a small amount of the food onto the inside of your wrist at bedtime and let it dry. (If the food is fairly solid add a little water to it and mash it up.) A red mark in the morning indicates an allergy.

The other method is longer and more complicated. It's based on the fact that your pulse increases in response to a problem food. You can feel your pulse at your wrist, at your neck to one side of your 'Adam's apple' or you could buy a cheap pulse rate monitor.

Step 1. Take your pulse when you're still in bed just after waking, just before each meal, at 30, 60 and 90 minutes after each meal, and just before you go to bed, *always at rest*. Don't eat between meals. That will make 14 readings (assuming three meals a day). In a notebook record the time of each reading and the reading itself, the time of each meal and the complete contents of the meal.

Step 2. After three days analyse the results. The difference between the various at-rest readings should be no more than 12 beats a minute. If the difference is higher a food problem should be suspected. Examine your food diary to see which foods are the most likely culprits.

Step 3. Test individual food suspects at the rate of one an hour, taking your pulse just before eating each one and again 30 minutes later. If your pulse after eating a food goes up by more than six beats a minute, or is more than 12 beats above your lowest pulse, you've probably identified a problem food.

▶ How do I know if I need an allergy/intolerance diet?

If you have irritable bowel symptoms then you very likely *do* have a food allergy or intolerance. The question is what sort of diet you should follow. If you have other symptoms in addition to your irritable bowel problems (for example, skin rashes, headaches or breathing difficulties) you may be better to approach the situation from the allergy/intolerance angle. If you don't have other symptoms then the low-fat, low-carbohydrate and IgG diets may be more productive.

▶ Can enzyme-rich foods help?

Enzymes are catalysts, that's to say, they speed up metabolic reactions, including the digestion of food, by millions of times. Without enzymes food would never get digested. Each type of food requires its own enzyme or enzymes. For example:

▶ Amylase digests carbohydrates such as starch and sugar.

▶ Cellulase breaks down fibre.

▶ Lactase digests milk sugar in dairy products.

▶ Lipase digests fat.

▶ Maltase converts complex sugars from grains into glucose.

▶ Phytase helps with digestion generally and is important for B vitamins.

▶ Protease digests proteins.

▶ Sucrase digests most sugars.

If you're deficient in a certain enzyme then eating the food on which it works is guaranteed to produce discomfort at the very least and possibly bloating, pain, nausea and diarrhoea. So could enzyme deficiency be the key to IBS? In Step 2 we looked at the role of enzyme supplements. Here we're going to look at the enzymes that occur naturally in food.

The first point to make about food is that heating to as little as 47° C inactivates most enzymes and boiling point is thought to destroy all of them. So it has to be fresh raw food. The second point is that enzymes are proteins and are destroyed by acid in the stomach. The question then is: do any enzymes survive in sufficient quantities to make a difference to the digestive process?

The answer to that question is that nobody really knows. Dr Edward Howell, whom we met in Step 2, spent years researching enzymes. He claimed that after raw food had been well-chewed in the mouth, it could spend 30 to 45 minutes in the upper part of the stomach unmixed with gastric juice. That is certainly true. He further claimed that during that period the enzymes in the raw food continued the process of digestion that had begun in the mouth. Whether that happens to any significant extent remains controversial. In fact, most mainstream nutritionists believe that 90 per cent of digestion occurs in the small intestine. Do any enzymes in food make it that far?

It's worth pointing out that human colostrum and breast milk contain at least 70 different enzymes with weird names such as alkaline phosphatise, amylase, lactate dehydrogenase, lactoperoxidase, transaminases and xanthine oxidase. It's possible they are there for some other reason but it seems probable they benefit the baby and do survive the infant stomach. In all probability some enzymes in food do get through in adults as well. If you can tolerate them, raw foods are certainly worth trying.

Those high in natural enzymes include:

Avocados	Grapes
Bananas	Honey (raw)
Coconut oil (extra virgin)	Kiwis

Mangos	Pineapples
Olive oil (extra virgin)	Sprouted seeds and legumes (probably the highest of all).
Papayas	

Key idea

In general you'll get more nutrients from cooked food than raw food. So eat some raw food every day but don't make it the mainstay of your diet.

Remember this

A 1991 study (Laugier R, Bernard JP, Berthezene P, Dupuy P) found that enzyme secretion by the pancreas declines with age. So it's important to try to boost your digestive enzymes as you get older.

▶ Can probiotic and prebiotic foods help?

We looked at probiotic and prebiotic supplements in Step 2. Here we're looking at foods that are naturally high in probiotics, and in a moment we'll also look at natural prebiotics. Remember that probiotics are defined as live microorganisms which when administered in adequate amounts confer a health benefit on the host. As with enzymes there's a question mark over the extent to which they can survive stomach acids. Most scientists, however, accept that some get through, even if it's only a tiny proportion. And it makes sense that some must, otherwise no one would ever have an upset caused by bacteria.

Here are some of the best probiotic sources:

▶ Live-cultured yoghurt containing *Lactobacilli* and *Bifidobacteria*, especially goat's milk yoghurt (but not those brands with artificial flavours or sweeteners or corn syrup)

▶ Kefir, a fermented drink made by adding kefir grains to milk – but it can also be made with water. In one study of people who were lactose intolerant, kefir reduced by half the flatulence caused by consuming milk or milk products. The bacteria in kefir vary according to the production method but typically it contains *Lactobacillus lacti, Lactobacillus rhamnosus, Bifidobacterium longum, Bifidobacterium breve, Lactobacillus acidophilus, Saccharomyces florentinus, Streptococcus diacetylactis, Leuconostoc cremoris, Lactobacillus plantarum* and *Lactobacillus case.*

▶ Microalgae such as spirulina, chorella and blue-green algae

▶ Miso (fermented barley, beans, rice or rye) and tempeh (fermented soya)

▶ Sauerkraut (fermented cabbage) provided it's unpasteurized and uncooked.

Raw, uncooked sauerkraut and kefir are especially interesting as they're good sources of *Lactobacillus plantarum*. In various studies *Lactobacillus plantarum*:

▶ reduced bloating, flatulence, intestinal pain and both constipation and diarrhoea in IBS patients

▶ reduced inflammation in the bowel

▶ boosted the immune system

▶ helped digest starch, protein, milk and milk products.

In addition, sauerkraut provides:

▶ Vitamins B and K

▶ Calcium, magnesium, folate, iron, potassium, copper and manganese

▶ The antioxidants lutein and zeaxanthin which are thought to be good for the eyes

▶ The antioxidants glutathione and superoxide dismustase

▶ Isothiocyanates which are believed to be protective against cancer.

For the first day or so sauerkraut may actually increase bloating, flatulence and diarrhoea, but the symptoms usually improve as the body adjusts. Another problem with sauerkraut is that it's high in tyramine which can cause migraine in sensitive individuals. And if you have thyroid problems consult with your doctor before eating sauerkraut on a regular basis.

PREBIOTIC FOODS

Prebiotics are non-digestible ingredients that provide food for probiotics. They were first identified and named only in 1995 and comprise:

▶ Inulin

▶ Galactooligosaccharides (GOS), also known as trans-galactooligosaccharides (TOS)

▶ Fructooligosaccharides (FOS)

▶ Lactulose, a synthetic sugar also known as galactofructose.

Most experts recommend around 6 g a day, which can be provided by:

Raw chicory root	9.3 g
Raw Jerusalem artichoke	19.0 g
Raw dandelion greens	24.7 g
Raw garlic	34.3 g
Raw leek	51.3 g
Raw onion	69.8 g
Cooked onion	120.0 g
Raw asparagus	120.0 g
Raw wheat bran	120.0 g
Wholewheat flour, cooked	125.0 g
Raw banana	600.0 g

Source: Moshfegh AJ, Friday JE, Goldman JP, Ahuja JK.

Not many people would want to eat a couple of raw garlic cloves a day, or raw Jerusalem artichoke. In practical terms, then, cooked onions, bananas and wholewheat products provide the best sources.

Ideally, prebiotics would feed only the 'good' bacteria. Unfortunately, that's not always the case. In fact, fructooligosaccharides (FOS) are specifically ruled out under the FODMAP diet (see above). Galactooligosaccharides (GOS) are a better bet because 'good' bacteria such *Bifidobacteria* and *Lactobacilli* are the first to feed on them, and they produce little or no gas. Although an excess intake of GOS could theoretically leave food over for the 'bad' bacteria, there aren't many natural sources. Soya beans are one of the few (but they're ruled out under some IBS diets) and GOS is mainly found in commercial preparations.

In general, you don't really want to increase your intake of prebiotics until you've (a) checked for SIBO and, if positive, eliminated it and (b) achieved a healthier balance of bacteria in your gut.

How should I eat?

It's clear you shouldn't carry on eating until you feel uncomfortable. If you do, the expansion of your stomach contents as they absorb gastric juice will take you beyond uncomfortable to extremely and even painfully bloated. Also, any movements that tend to squash a full stomach (such as bending down) can cause stomach acid to be squeezed up into the oesophagus, causing heartburn. Most of all, a full stomach is likely to trigger defecation which, if you suffer from IBS-D, you may not want. So it's best never to feel full.

For this reason, some nutritionists recommend having more frequent, smaller meals – four, five or six a day. That can be good advice. On the other hand, it's when the stomach is empty that the migrating motor complex (MMC – see above) flushes bacteria and any remaining food particles out of the small intestine. If the stomach is seldom empty there will be fewer of these waves and too many bacteria may remain. So this is something to experiment with.

It's certainly good advice to chew food well and to eat calmly sitting at a table so as to avoid swallowing air. However, swallowed air doesn't contribute much to bloating as most of it is eliminated by belching.

Have plenty to drink. The digestive tract needs enormous quantities of liquid. If your urine is a pale straw colour then you're having enough.

Making sense of it all

So you've now read about an anti-inflammatory diet, a low-fat diet, various low-carbohydrate diets, an IgG diet, allergy/intolerance diets and more. It can all seem quite bewildering. You may be looking at the long lists of restricted foods and thinking, 'What's left that I *can* eat?' In fact you'll find there's plenty.

The first thing to say is that the causes of irritable bowel symptoms are highly individual. Just because one IBS sufferer can eat a certain thing doesn't mean you can. It's a point well underlined by the IBS Research Appeal which asked 322 female and 78 male long-term IBS sufferers which foods helped their symptoms and which made them worse. Here are the results and if you look closely you'll see that some foods appear on both lists. For example, citrus fruit was thought to be the sixth most helpful food but was also the fourth most avoided.

THE TOP 20 MOST HELPFUL FOODS ACCORDING TO IBS SUFFERERS

1	Fish	11	Bran
2	Green vegetables	12	Bananas
3	Other vegetables	13	Chicken
4	Non-citrus fruit	14	Bland foods
5	Rice	15	Salad
6	Citrus fruit	16	Potatoes
7	Brown bread	17	White bread
8	Yoghurt	18	Porridge
9	Cereals	19	Apricots, dates, figs & prunes
10	Pasta	20	Biscuits

THE TOP 20 MOST AVOIDED FOODS BY IBS SUFFERERS

1	Spicy foods	7	Cereals
2	Fried and fatty foods	8	Non-citrus fruit
3	Greens	9	Chocolate
4	Citrus fruit	10	Bran
5	Cheese	11	Pulses (beans, lentils etc)
6	Onions and leeks	12	Vegetables (non-green)

13	Brown bread	17	Beef
14	Salad	18	White bread
15	Nuts	19	Eggs
16	Sweets and desserts	20	Dairy products

Nevertheless, there are some very significant generalizations that can be made, which I call Phase 1:

▶ Very few IBS sufferers can tolerate grains or tubers, so definitely eliminate those.

▶ The majority of IBS sufferers have problems with lactose, so eliminate dairy as well.

▶ A significant proportion of IBS suffers can't handle fructose without glucose, so eliminate those foods, too (see the list of excess fructose foods in the SIBO section above).

▶ A significant proportion of IBS sufferers have problems with fat so cut it right down.

▶ Everyone, not just IBS sufferers, will benefit from an anti-inflammatory diet.

Those five things should make a huge difference to most IBS sufferers. Note that lactose and fructose intolerance may not be permanent problems. If you have SIBO and clear it successfully then you may be able to eat those food groups again.

In addition, whatever diet you follow, under Phase 1 you should also avoid:

▶ Alcohol

▶ Coffee and other caffeinated drinks

▶ Decaffeinated coffee

▶ Carbonated drinks

▶ Olestra (a fat substitute with the brand name Olean)

▶ Sorbitol, which is both an artificial sweetener (as used, for example, in sugarless gum, dietetic jam and dietetic chocolate) and occurs naturally in significant quantities in apple juice, apricots, dates, peaches, pears, plums and dried fruit. About half of adults experience problems with 10 g of sorbitol, for example, and some have problems with as little as 5 g. (As a polyol, sorbitol is excluded under the FODMAPS diet.)

▶ Garlic – although it has important benefits, garlic is a frequent cause of upsets in IBS sufferers. (It's ruled out under both the FODMAPS and IgG diets.) Bacteria in your gut can feed on the fructan of garlic causing gas, and the digested material can then attract water, causing diarrhoea. Watch out for it in processed foods.

▶ Processed foods (as far as possible) – there can be so many different ingredients that it becomes almost impossible to keep track of them. Keep it simple by sticking to fresh foods as much as you can.

If that works, great. When your IBS symptoms are resolved you can try reintroducing these things, if you wish, to see how you get on.

If it doesn't work, or only brings about a mild improvement, you're going to have to move on to Phase 2 which gets a lot more scientific:

▶ Analyse your food diary. As recommended at the start of the chapter, you should be recording *everything* that goes down your throat every day, including medicines, together with your irritable bowel symptoms and your bowel movements. Everything must be given a time and it's essential you write clearly so you can pick up things with a quick sweep of the eye. Use different coloured highlighters to draw attention to different suspect foods. If you uncover a connection between irritable bowel symptoms and a certain food, eliminate that food.

▶ Eliminate foods that appear in all the low-carbohydrate diets and the IgG diet. You'll see that there's a considerable overlap between GAPS, FODMAPS and IgG so it's not as formidable as it sounds. If there's a substantial improvement, continue with this 'combined diet' but reintroduce foods at the rate of one every four days, gradually increasing the 'dose' up to a normal portion. If your symptoms worsen you'll know not to eat that food any more. If your symptoms remain stable with the reintroduced food you know you can safely continue to eat it.

▶ If you get only a mild improvement with the 'combined diet' then it suggests you need a diet that will eliminate bacteria in the small intestine more rapidly. In that case ask your doctor for a SIBO test and if it's positive go onto the elemental diet.

▶ While all of this is going on, you should investigate the possibility that an allergy or intolerance is part or all of the problem. If you have symptoms in addition to irritable bowel symptoms then (as described above) an allergy/intolerance should be suspected. Examine your food diary to see if you can spot a connection between certain foods, your irritable bowel symptoms and those additional symptoms. If so, avoid those foods and introduce the measures to tackle the cause of the allergy/intolerance.

Remember this

When you've discovered a diet that works for you it's vital you stick with it, even when you're feeling fine. It's tough not being able to eat some lovely dish that everyone else is enjoying but, unfortunately, that's the nature of an irritable bowel. Many sufferers relapse simply because they eat something they know they shouldn't. So treat yourself to 'tough love' at all times and be disciplined.

Focus points

1 Fat can cause your gut to spasm – you may need to reduce your intake.
2 'Bad' bacteria are a cause of irritable bowel symptoms.
3 Those 'bad' bacteria are nourished by certain foods that you eat.
4 You can reduce 'bad' bacteria and increase 'good' bacteria by changing your diet.
5 You could also have a food intolerance caused by a lack of certain enzymes – again a change of diet will help.

Next step

In this chapter we've looked at the way certain foods can cause irritable bowel symptoms and the possible diets for avoiding those problems. In the next chapter we'll be coming at the situation from a different direction. We'll be looking at ways of stopping your digestive tract from reacting as it does.

5

Step 5: Take control of your brains

In this chapter you will learn:

▶ *How your gut has a 'brain' of its own*

▶ *How a nervous system malfunction may cause irritable bowel symptoms*

▶ *How you can use hypnotic techniques to take conscious control of unconscious processes.*

Because IBS was once something of a mystery illness, and because sufferers were often depressed, doctors began prescribing antidepressants. Tricyclic antidepressants, it so happens, can slow down bowel movements. They also reduce certain kinds of pain. So they were often successful in treating IBS and that success seemed to confirm to many health professionals that IBS was 'all in the mind'.

Well, it isn't.

It's really not surprising if irritable bowel sufferers are depressed. But it's usually the irritable bowel that causes the depression, not the other way around. Nevertheless, there is an amazing link between the mind and the gut, which has to be taken into account.

In Step 5 you're going to be learning how to take conscious control of what would normally be unconscious processes. Almost certainly the 'automatic pilot' that should run your digestive system efficiently has suffered a malfunction. You're going to learn to override it.

Back in the mists of time there were no central nervous systems. Tubular animals stuck to rocks and waited for food to pass. They were, in a sense, just stomachs and their 'brain' functions were largely to do with the stomach. That's why you and I today still have a 'brain' in our digestive tracts.

This 'brain', known as the enteric nervous system (ENS), has something like 100 million nerve cells and produces large quantities of neurotransmitters, including at least 90 per cent of the body's serotonin (a hormone that regulates mood, sleep, learning and constriction of the blood vessels). So you actually have two 'brains' and although the ENS can function independently, they communicate with one another via the vagus nerve.

That vagus connection means both 'brains' can influence your intestines. Something in that system has gone wrong somewhere. With our present knowledge we don't know what exactly but that doesn't stop us consciously putting the system back on track.

In fact we all know how our thoughts and emotions affect the gut. The connection is reflected in our everyday speech. We talk about having a 'gut instinct'. We say we have 'butterflies in the tummy'. And, indeed, even those with normal bowels can have an attack of diarrhoea in a stressful situation. Those are all normal effects of the 'two brain axis'.

There are three reasons it's vitally important to work on these 'brains' when it comes to an irritable bowel:

▶ Something is going wrong somewhere in the parts of the nervous system that handle peristalsis and pain sensitivity in the gut.

▶ Stress exacerbates irritable bowel symptoms so stress has to be controlled.

▶ The symptoms can create a fear which intensifies the perception of pain.

So let's see how much your 'brains' are involved in your irritable bowel.

Diagnostic test

1 Do your irritable bowel symptoms get worse when you're under stress or improve when you're very relaxed (on holiday, for example)?

   a No
   b Yes

2 Do you feel sick, or actually vomit, when you're apprehensive about something?

   a No
   b Yes

3 Have you any reason to believe you were abused in childhood, or have you been abused as an adult?

   a No
   b Yes

4 Have you ever suffered from low moods or depression?

   a No
   b Yes

5 Do you suffer from any of backache, musculoskeletal (MSK) pain, fatigue, nausea, urinary problems or gynaecological problems?

   a No
   b Yes

6 My intestinal pain is:

   a infrequent, short-lived and quite manageable.
   b often present and occasionally quite severe.
   c almost constant and quite unbearable.

7 How would you describe yourself?

   a Calm and tranquil
   b Always on edge
   c Angry

8 My blood pressure is:

   a normal for my age.
   b a bit high for my age.
   c very high – I'm on medication to control it.

9 I find it:

   a easy to relax.
   b only possible to relax when everything has been done.
   c almost impossible to relax.

10 I sleep:

   a soundly and awake ready for the day.
   b fitfully and awake feeling tired.
   c very badly – I suffer from insomnia.

Your score:

In some cases stress may cause an irritable bowel and in all cases it exacerbates it. If you mostly answered 'yes' for questions one to five, and if you mostly answered 'b' or 'c' for questions six to ten, then

The toothpaste tube

You know how it is. You carefully squeeze the toothpaste tube from the bottom but then somebody else comes along, squeezes it in the middle and forces the toothpaste down to the wrong end. It's a bit like that with your irritable gut.

In order for food to pass through your 'processing plant' your gut has to be squeezed in an intelligent sequence. Otherwise, as with the toothpaste, the food will end up going backwards instead of forwards. Those contractions, out of sequence, can cause pain. Sometimes a lot of pain.

Something has to be directing those contractions. Something quite clever. We don't yet know exactly how it all works, but bit by bit the jigsaw is being pieced together. Have you ever wondered, for example, how it is that the contractions of your rectum cease when all the matter in it has been evacuated? Research has shown that it's to do with nerves in the anal canal and sphincters. Once they stop sensing the passage of waste matter they signal the rectum to cease its contractions. At least, that's what normally happens. In some IBS sufferers that mechanism malfunctions and the rectum goes on contracting when it shouldn't, sometimes quite painfully.

Somehow we have to speak to the 'brain' that's directing the contractions and re-educate it. That's what you'll be learning to do in this Step.

In 1992, a team led by Professor Peter Whorwell, a pioneer of gut-directed hypnotherapy (see below), published a paper in the *Lancet* (the world's leading general medical journal) proving the connection between emotion and the speed with which waste moved through the large intestine. The team found that anger and excitement both increased speed (as well as pulse and respiration rate) while happiness reduced it.

Another study, at University Hospitals, Dusseldorf, this time on rats, found that, under stress, while the processing of food by the stomach was actually delayed, and transit time through the small intestine decreased only by about one-third the speed through the large intestine dramatically accelerated, reducing transit from more than 15 hours to under one and a half hours. The researchers stated that the effects appeared similar to stress-induced diarrhoea in humans. As to the precise mechanism, that remains controversial, but some researchers believe corticotrophin releasing factor (CRF), a neurotransmitter secreted by the hypothalamus in response to stress, is the key.

Other research has pinpointed at least one area of the brain where there's a problem in IBS. Functional magnetic resonance imaging (MRI) and positron emission tomography (PET) have consistently shown that the processing of painful stimuli in the part of the brain known as the anterior cingulate cortex is exaggerated.

Stress, then, is especially bad for IBS sufferers as well as for health generally. When you're stressed, among other things:

▶ stress hormones are released into the blood

▶ blood pressure rises

▶ heart rate increases

▶ sugar and fat pour into the bloodstream, depositing plaque in your arteries

▶ your muscles, including those that control the gut, become tense

▶ transit through the large intestine is dramatically accelerated

▶ pain signals are exaggerated.

So even if stress was not the cause of your irritable bowel, it will certainly make it a whole lot worse. In addition, stress causes a long list of health problems ranging from heartburn, headaches and allergies up to diabetes, heart disease and cancer. So in this Step you'll also be learning to relax.

Gut-directed hypnotherapy

Here's a statistic that may astonish you. Between 30 and 40 per cent of IBS sufferers enjoy significant improvement in their symptoms when treated with a ... placebo. In other words, an inert sugar pill. Even more astounding, placebo outperformed almost every other IBS treatment in one study, *even though the patients knew it was a placebo*.

This tells us something very important about IBS. It confirms that the mind plays a role. And when you understand that your gut has a 'brain' which is connected to the brain in your head it's not so surprising.

Let me emphasize right now that the success of the placebo does not mean that an irritable bowel is all in the mind. It simply underlines the fact that there's a malfunction somewhere in the nervous system and that being given the placebo somehow helps some sufferers to take better control of their 'brains' and engage their natural healing abilities.

The best way we know of tackling that kind of problem is not a scalpel but gut-directed hypnotherapy. In fact, it's the world's most powerful irritable bowel treatment so far. Using it in combination with standard therapies such as antispasmodics, Professor Whorwell and his team, working in Manchester, England, have achieved a success rate (that's to say, a substantial decrease in symptoms) of 70 per cent. One to five years after treatment ended, 83 per cent of those who responded were still doing well.

In physiological terms, gut-directed hypnotherapy can:

▶ alter the gut's response to food

▶ influence gastric acid secretion and gastric (stomach) emptying

▶ slow transit time from the mouth to the beginning of the large intestine

▶ reduce the strength of contractions in the large intestine

▶ reduce the perception of pain in the gut

▶ reduce the microscopic inflammation that's present

▶ boost the immune system.

And the power of gut-directed hypnotherapy doesn't stop there. It also has an impact on associated symptoms such as:

► Heartburn

► Anxiety and depression

► Fibromyalgia

► Non-cardiac chest pain.

On television you may have seen hypnotized volunteers apparently believing themselves to be naked, or in love with a chair, or even floating above a stage without apparent support. Unfortunately, the real-life results achieved by hypnosis are seldom as dramatic or as quick. Professor Whorwell and his team offer a one-hour session each week for 12 weeks. It's their experience that patients who haven't responded by then never will. (In which case, they are then offered other therapies.) In between sessions, patients have to do a little daily homework, listening to recordings. So although there are only 12 hours with the therapist in person, there's a total of 84 hours of therapy.

Don't be disappointed if you don't get the immediate results stage hypnotism may have led you to expect. In the real world these things take time.

The first two sessions will probably be for general relaxation. It's from the third session onwards that things usually become more specific. You might be asked to imagine healing energy flowing into your abdomen from your hand, for example. Or you might be asked to visualize your digestive system as a smoothly flowing river. Gradually you'll increase your ability to calm your digestive tract.

There's one big drawback with gut-directed hypnotherapy. It's this. There just aren't enough skilled hypnotherapists who are trained to deal with irritable bowels. In the UK, for example, there's a Register of IBS hypnotherapists which, at the time of writing, comprised just 130 names. Given that each hypnotherapist can only handle something like 150 patients a year, that's merely scratching the surface of the problem. The alternative is to buy hypnotherapy on CDs or … to hypnotize yourself.

Key idea

The first thing is to believe that you do have power over your gut. That's important. And, indeed, you do know it because you only have to think of something horrible to experience that churning in your stomach. That's the proof.

SELF-HYPNOSIS FOR IBS

In April 1845, Dr James Esdaile was operating on a man with a swollen testicle. The procedure was particularly painful and this was two years before the Scottish obstetrician James Young Simpson discovered the anaesthetic qualities of chloroform. Dr Esdaile turned to his assistant and asked if he knew anything about Mesmerism, the name then used for what we now call hypnotism.

'I have a great mind to try it on this man,' said Dr Esdaile, 'but as I never saw it practised, and know it only from reading, I shall probably not succeed.'

He did try it, he did succeed and he went on to complete many more operations using hypnosis.

So it can't be that difficult.

And it's not. In fact, all hypnosis is actually self-hypnosis You can't actually be hypnotized by someone else. You can go to see a hypnotherapist and be led by that person into trance. But the hypnotherapist can't *make* you hypnotized. You do that yourself. Which means you can very effectively use self-hypnosis at home for your irritable bowel (and many other things).

What is hypnosis? Derren Brown, the TV mentalist, says he doesn't know what hypnotism really is himself. What we can say for sure is that it's an altered state of consciousness or, more specifically, a state of consciousness that's different to what we consider to be our normal waking state. In other words, a trance.

We all go into trances every day. When you're totally absorbed in a book or a newspaper and unaware of the things going on around you you're in a trance. It's as simple as that. When you swing a golf club or throw a dart and get almost exactly the result you want you're in a trance. When you're making love with your partner you're in a trance.

So let's get started on your first session.

 Try it now

Step 1. Get yourself comfortable in a place you won't be disturbed. It's not a good idea to lie on the bed because you might fall asleep. But you could sit up on the bed supported by pillows, or arrange yourself in a comfortable chair.

Step 2. Decide the length of time you wish to spend in self-hypnosis. Initially I'd suggest 15 minutes. That should give you enough time to achieve a deep state of trance without feeling anxiety about 'wasting' time or needing to get on with something else. As you get used to self-hypnosis and employ more complicated visualizations you can increase the time. So, having got comfortable, you should say something like this: 'I am now going to hypnotize myself for 15 minutes'. You might like to append the actual time by adding '… which means I will come out of self-hypnosis at 19.30 (or whatever)'.

Step 3. This is a key step because it's where you state the purpose of your hypnosis. Initially you should just focus on inducing a state of deep relaxation. In later sessions, when you're more proficient, you can go on to tackle your irritable bowel symptoms more specifically. So for your first session you could say something like this:

> I am entering into a state of self-hypnosis so that I can hand over to my unconscious mind the task of inducing a state of deep relaxation.

The exact words aren't important but make sure you say you're inviting your *unconscious* to deal with the matter. In later sessions you can tackle your irritable bowel more directly by saying, for example:

> I am entering into a state of self-hypnosis so that I can hand over to my unconscious mind the task of curing my diarrhoea (or constipation, as the case may be).

> I am entering into a trance for the purpose of allowing my unconscious mind to make the adjustments that will reduce my irritable bowel symptoms.

I am entering into a trance to allow my unconscious to stop me being fearful about **my irritable bowel**.

Step 4. State how you want to feel when you come out of your trance. For example, for your first session you might say, 'As I come out of my trance I will feel incredibly relaxed'. In later sessions you might say, 'As I come out of trance my symptoms will get better and better and better'. (According to Professor Whorwell, saying things three times is more effective than saying them once or twice.)

Step 5. This is the actual process of self-hypnosis. Basically you're going to engage in turn your three main representational systems (sight, hearing, touch) to bring the trance about. In the first part of the process you will be noting things you can actually see, hear and feel *in the room where you are*. In the second part you will be noting things you can see, hear and feel *in an imaginary scene*.

In this process, some people talk to themselves internally but I recommend that *you say everything out loud*. For that reason you'll want to be in a private place. You might imagine that you'd 'wake' yourself up but, in fact, the sound of your own voice, done the right way, will intensify the effect. (If, however, speaking out loud doesn't work for you then by all means speak internally.)

a From your comfortable position look at some small thing in the room in front of you and say out loud what you are looking at. Choose things you can see without moving your head. For example, 'I am looking at the door handle'. Then, without rushing, focus on another small item. For example, 'I am now looking at a glass of water on the table'. Then move on to a third item. For example, 'I am looking at the light switch'. When you have your three visual references, move on to (b).

b Switch attention to sounds and, in the same way, note one after another until you have three, each time saying out loud what you're hearing. Then move on to (c).

c Note things that you can feel with your body. For example, you might say, 'I can feel the seat pressing against my buttocks'. When you have your three, move on.

d Now repeat steps (a) to (c) but with only two items for each sense, that's to say, two images, two sounds and two feelings. They must be *different* from the ones you used before. *Speak a little more slowly.*

e Again repeat steps (a) to (c) but with only one item per sense, that's to say, one image, one sound and one feeling. Again, they must be *different* from any that have gone before. *Speak even more slowly.*

f Close your eyes, if they're not already closed, and, for your first session, think of a relaxed scene. Keep it fairly simple. It might, for example, be you lying on a beautiful, sandy beach, the sun warming your skin, and the blue water rhythmically lapping on the shore in front of you. In later sessions you might visualize food moving steadily along through your gut like a smooth-flowing river (slower if you have diarrhoea, faster if you have constipation).

g Using your imagined scene, go through the same process you already used for the real scene, but beginning with just one example of each of the three senses, that is, one image, one sound and one feeling. For example, you might 'see' a seagull bobbing on the water, 'hear' the waves on the sand, and 'feel' the heat of the sun on your skin. When you've done that, increase to two examples and then three. (Three is usually enough, but if you've stipulated a lengthy session you may need to continue with your fantasy scene by going on to name four images, sounds and feelings, or five or even more.) Remember, each example must be *different*. You'll probably find you're automatically speaking very slowly now but, if not, make a point of *slowing your voice down more and more*.

h After the allotted time you should begin to come out of trance automatically. But it may help to announce, 'I'll count to three and when I reach three I'll be (whatever you said in (d))'. Don't worry about getting 'stuck' in a trance. That won't happen. You may feel a little woozy for a while. If so, don't drive a car or do anything demanding until you're sure you're okay to do so.

Remember this

Milton Erickson (1901–1980) was one of the most famous hypnotherapists of his era. As a boy he contracted polio and in his fifties he developed post-polio syndrome which caused muscle weakness and severe pain. He used self-hypnosis to keep the pain under control but even he, one of the most successful hypnotherapists of all time, had to repeat it every day. As he explained: 'It usually takes me an hour after I awaken to get all the pain out.' So don't expect a miracle after just one session. Go through the whole procedure every day for a couple of weeks before passing judgement. Hopefully you'll notice some improvement in that time. But, realistically, it may take up to three months of daily sessions to gain the full benefit of self-hypnosis. And you'll need to 'top-up' from time to time.

Key idea

Having completed a psychological procedure there's a natural tendency to check to see how the pain is afterwards. In other words, to focus on the pain. But as soon as you 'check to see if the pain has gone away' you cause it to intensify. Try not to do that.

Case study

'I was diagnosed with IBS about five years ago. I was getting caught short at least once a week, was frightened to go out unless I knew there was a toilet handy, and we'd had to cancel two family holidays to see relatives in Australia because I was too nervous about the toilet situation. A friend recommended gut-directed hypnotherapy and I was fortunate to be seen fairly quickly. I'm not sure how the hypnotherapy works but after just a few weekly visits I saw a great improvement. The hypnotherapist provided me with tapes to listen to between sessions and I played them every day. It took about a dozen sessions but I go back for top-ups from time to time. Apart from that, I'm not receiving any medical intervention. I now go months without any attack, although I occasionally do balloon out. But I can cope with that. The greatest thing recently was to be able to sit down to Christmas dinner with all the family.' Lily (29)

The gut to brain connection

Although in this Step we're mainly concerned with the way your 'brains' influence your gut, it's useful to understand to what extent your gut influences your brain and your mind. The neurologist

Dr Natasha Campbell-McBride sees a clear connection between mental disorders and digestive disorders. She believes that 'bad' bacteria in the gut produce dangerous toxins such as alcohol, its by-product acetaldehyde (believed to be responsible for hangovers), and opiate-like substances. There are children, she argues, who have never known anything other than a hangover-like state, due to dysbiosis (abnormal gut flora). In her book *Gut and Psychology Syndrome* (Medinform Publishing, 2010) she contends that 'most children and adults with learning disabilities, psychiatric disorders and allergies present with digestive problems'. Her GAPS diet (see Step 4), she believes, helps children with autism, ADHD/ADD, dyslexia, dyspraxia, depression and schizophrenia. None of that proves that things can work the other way around and that the brain can cause problems in the digestive tract. But it makes it a lot easier to believe.

Neuro-Linguistic Programming (NLP)

You don't actually have to go into a trance to reprogram your brain. There are other ways. Back in the 1970s, two young men called Richard Bandler and John Grinder, working with various specialists including Milton Erickson who was mentioned above, developed a whole family of techniques which they called Neuro-Linguistic Programming (NLP). Many people learn NLP from a qualified therapist, but I'm now going to teach you three NLP techniques you can begin using today. They should all help you combat stress and be more relaxed.

The first one we're interested in here is a sophisticated kind of visualization.

It works like this. When you visualize something you don't recreate it exactly as it is. That's impossible. Your feelings about the subject distort the imagined scene in various ways. For example, if I ask you to imagine being in hospital you'll possibly visualize a very drab scene, drained of colour, with the sounds of people groaning, the smell of ether, and the weight of the building seeming to press down on you. You won't like it. These qualities of visualizations are what's known in NLP as 'submodalities'.

But rather than allowing your emotions to dictate the submodalities you can turn everything back to front and choose the submodalities that will induce the emotions you would prefer to feel. To continue with the example of the hospital, I'm going to ask you to imagine that the walls are painted in vibrant colours and that your bedding is just like your bedding at home. Around you your fellow patients are all chuckling. In the air there's the smell of flowers. And the building has only one storey with large floor to ceiling windows through which you can see blue skies and a beautiful garden. Now you probably feel more positive about being in hospital.

Let's now apply this technique to your digestive tract.

Try it now

Step 1. Get yourself nicely relaxed somewhere comfortable – perhaps on the bed.

Step 2. Focus on an image of yourself at some time in the past when you were in perfect health and identify the submodalities that go with that image. Are the colours bright, for example? Is there music? Is the sun shining? Is your skin glowing? Is there a particular feeling in your body?

Step 3. Focus on your digestive tract. Visualize it working perfectly and, while doing so, make use of the submodalities you identified in Step 2. Turn them all up to the maximum. For example, if bright yellow is the colour you associate with perfect health then flood the image of your digestive tract with bright yellow light. If Albinoni's famous Adagio evokes the precise movement of a fine Swiss watch then play it loudly in your head as you 'see' your digestive tract calmly and smoothly moving the food along. If glowing skin epitomizes health then visualize the walls of your digestive tract dazzling you with their incandescence.

Step 4. Say something along the following lines: 'I am well and my wonderful digestive tract is completely healthy.' To reinforce the message you can go on to describe how calm, controlled and pain free it is.

Step 5. Repeat regularly.

Anchoring for relaxation

You know stress is bad for your irritable bowel symptoms. You know you get more nervous than you should in certain situations. But try as you might, you just *can't* relax.

Wouldn't it be wonderful if there was some kind of button you could press that would automatically *make* you relaxed? Well, there is something that comes close. It's an NLP technique known as 'anchoring'.

An anchor is a development of the conditioned stimulus described by Ivan Pavlov (1849–1936) in his famous work on the training of dogs. He used a metronome to call dogs to their food and, very soon, the dogs began salivating in response to the metronome. They couldn't help it. The behaviour had become automatic. Most people are not very astonished to learn of Pavlov's findings. It's what would be expected. Nevertheless, his research has significant implications for you in learning to relax. In the same way that salivating had become automatic for the dogs, so relaxing could become automatic for you.

Anchoring is NLP's version of Pavlov's conditioned stimulus. And, in fact, whether you realize it or not, you already respond to anchors. A certain piece of music might always make you feel romantic because it was playing when you first met the person you're in love with. The smell of coffee might make you feel warm and gregarious because you associate it with the friendly bustle of a certain café. And the mere sight of a comedian making a trademark gesture might make you laugh, not because the gesture itself is funny but because it's an anchor that recalls all the previous times the comedian made you laugh.

CHOOSING ANCHORS

To give the best possible chance of success, your anchor should meet the following conditions:

▶ It should be as natural and logical as possible.

▶ It should be something to which you'd normally *want* to respond.

▶ It should be easy to activate, but not to activate accidentally.

▶ It should involve two or preferably three senses.

Try it now

Step 1. Choose your anchors. I'm going to suggest you stroke your chin and whisper the word 'relax', thus involving the optimum three senses:

▶ A visual anchor – the sight of your hand coming up to your face and moving in front of your chin.

▶ An audible anchor – the sound of your voice whispering 'relax' and the sound of your fingers against the skin of your face.

▶ A kinaesthetic anchor – the feeling of your fingers against the skin of your face.

Step 2. Think of a time when you felt truly serene, calm, imperturbable and, above all, relaxed. However, if you really can't remember such a time then recall a film in which someone you admire was really 'laid back'. Identify the submodalities that are associated with relaxation. (If you've forgotten about submodalities see above.)

Step 3. Revel in that feeling of relaxation. See, hear, touch, taste and smell everything to do with relaxation. Make the sensation as powerful as possible by turning up those submodalities as far as they'll go.

Step 4. Just *before* your feeling of relaxation reaches its peak, set your anchors by gently stroking your chin and whispering the word 'relax'.

Step 5. Repeat steps 1–4 several times.

Step 6. Visualize a scene that normally makes you anxious but, on this occasion, see yourself being incredibly relaxed. In NLP this is known as 'future pacing'. If you can feel relaxed while contemplating the scene then the anchor is starting to work.

Step 7. As soon as possible, deliberately seek out a situation that will test your ability to relax. Fire your anchors. Over the next few days, keep on experiencing demanding situations and keep on firing your anchors. You'll need to deal successfully with maybe a score of situations before the anchor will become permanent and automatic.

Remember this

The setting of anchors can be quite an art. As I emphasized in Step 4, you need to do it just *before* the emotion you're dealing with reaches peak intensity. In that way, the anchor will be associated with strong and growing emotion. If you set your anchor *after* peak emotion then it will be associated with a decline in feeling, which is not the result you want at all. The anchor also needs to be 'pure'. In other words, if you're, say, feeling sceptical when you try this procedure then you'll be anchoring relaxation contaminated with scepticism – again, not the result you want.

Key idea

The more you use an anchor, the more powerful it becomes. We're all familiar with the way sportsmen, say, punch the air or do a little dance when they've scored. What they're doing is 'stacking' an anchor. Each time they perform that ritual they, as it were, add the power of that new victory to all the previous victories. That, in turn, creates the psychological impression of an unstoppable momentum of success. You can do just the same with relaxation.

Discrediting an inner voice

We all have an inner voice and precisely because it is 'inner' we tend to attach great importance to it. But, in fact, there's no reason this inner voice should be any more right than your conscious voice.

You know how it is. You have to, say, give a speech. Logically, you know you're perfectly capable of speaking. You've been doing it since you were two. Yet there's that inner voice telling you something like this: 'Everyone is going to be bored by you. They'll think you're a complete idiot. They'll probably walk out.' As a result you get an attack of diarrhoea.

Well, don't let your inner voice faze you. Richard Bandler says he often shouts at his inner voice, 'Shut up!'

That can work quite well. But rather than simply trying to shout down your negative inner voice, a more effective method is to *discredit* it. Right now it probably sounds authoritative. But what if it were to sound like the voice of the politician you most distrust, or a cartoon character? Then maybe you wouldn't take such notice of it.

Try it now

Step 1. Think of a person you greatly distrust. It could be someone you know, it could be a contemporary politician or it could be a historical figure such as Hitler. Hear that person's voice and identify what qualities (submodalities) in the voice make you distrustful. Is there something about the pitch, perhaps? The rhythm? The timbre?

Step 2. Now think of the negative thing your inner voice has been telling you, but instead of hearing the usual voice, hear instead the distrusted voice, complete with all those unreliable, cheating, lying submodalities. Really enter into this experience. See the face of that distrusted person and realize that you don't believe a word they're saying. It may be helpful to play some music in your head, perhaps something that comes from a satirical programme or which somehow symbolizes indomitable opposition (if you're familiar with it, the Colonel Bogey March works well).

Step 3. Now push that distrusted voice and its distrusted, negative message further and further away from you until it gets fainter and fainter and you can't hear it any more.

Step 4. Check to see how you now feel. Hopefully a lot less negative.

Step 5. Visualize a scene in the future in which you behave in the way you want and successfully do the very thing your negative voice had been telling you that you couldn't do. That will help you install the new behaviour in your unconscious.

Step 6. Actually *do* the thing your negative voice had been telling you that you couldn't do.

Biofeedback

Biofeedback is another way of re-educating your 'brains' and, if you can't find a suitable hypnotherapist, you might have the luck to discover a good specialist in biofeedback. The essence of biofeedback is to make the normally invisible processes of the body visible. To a certain extent you can then learn to take conscious control of them.

Breathing is a very clear example of a normally unconscious process over which you can take conscious control. For that you don't need any clever biofeedback technology, because you can sense and hear your own breathing. But you can't normally sense very much about what's going on in your gut. That's where technology is starting to help.

If you opt for biofeedback, your therapist will connect sensors to your body so you can see what's happening with various bodily functions on a monitor or series of read-outs. You'll learn to spot the things that are contributing to your irritable bowel symptoms and, with the help of the therapist, learn to modify your bodily functions through the relaxation of muscles and other techniques. For example, using anorectal manometry it's possible to see how much pressure you're able to create to evacuate your bowels. You can learn to increase it if it's weak, or how to relax the sphincter if it's over-tightened.

So does it work? The research is generally positive. In a study conducted at the Royal North Shore Hospital, Sydney, Australia, for example, 25 women suffering from IBS with pelvic floor dyssynergia were given anorectal feedback therapy. Pelvic floor dyssynergia means the muscles and ligaments of the pelvic floor no longer work in a co-ordinated fashion. The women were taught how to relax and use their abdominal muscles and also practised expelling a water-filled balloon. After three months of weekly sessions, three-quarters of the women rated themselves 'improved' or 'very improved'. A similar study conducted at Chulalongkorn University, Bangkok, achieved a success rate of 60 per cent.

More relaxation therapies

Hypnotherapy, NLP visualization and biofeedback are ways of getting directly at the malfunctions in your 'brains'. It's also worth trying to come at your irritable bowel problems indirectly, by learning to relax, by mastering stressful situations and, quite simply, by being happier. As we've seen, hormonal and muscular changes associated with anxiety and unhappiness may not cause IBS but they certainly are behind most of the periodic flare-ups.

In a study of 80 IBS sufferers conducted by the Department of Psychosomatic Medicine and Psychotherapy at the University of Munich, half were taught relaxation techniques and half were given the standard treatment plus two counselling interviews. The researchers concluded that relaxation was 'significantly superior' both immediately and at the three-month follow-up. So let's take a look at some relaxation and anti-stress techniques, beginning with cognitive therapy (CT).

Cognitive therapy

In the 1960s, Dr Aaron Beck at the University of Pennsylvania School of Medicine developed a very powerful system for combating low moods. He had noticed that patients suffering from depression had a much lower opinion of themselves and their achievements than they should. A man who had climbed several of the world's 8,000-metre plus peaks would describe himself as a failure because he hadn't reached the summit of K2. A woman who could speak five languages would dismiss her linguistic skills on the grounds that 'everyone in my family speaks at least five'. The mother of three healthy, happy, successful children would lament that she was a 'terrible mum' because her home-made cakes were inedible. He concluded that it was people's cognitions (thoughts) about events in their lives, rather than the events themselves, that affected their mental state, so he called his system 'cognitive therapy' (in its widest application also known as 'cognitive behavioural therapy').

You can learn CT with a trained psychotherapist. You can also try it on yourself. That's what I'm going to explain to you right now.

You could say that people who always remain positive and optimistic are naturals at CT, while those who get depressed are not. But CT is more than a treatment for depression. It's also a treatment for anxiety, stress and unhappiness in general. Which means it can be used to alleviate the irritable bowel symptoms that are exacerbated by those emotions.

Dr Beck identified ten different kinds of negative thinking. There isn't space to go into all of them here so I'll just focus on the ones that are most likely to contribute to irritable bowel problems.

PERFECTIONISM

Do you strive so hard for perfection that you find it difficult to complete any task? And afterwards, do you torture yourself with the thought that what you did wasn't good enough? If so, you're causing yourself a lot of distress for nothing. And that distress can manifest itself as irritable bowel symptoms.

The fact is, there's no such thing as perfection and it's pointless striving for it. Of course be conscientious, meticulous and painstaking. In many jobs these are essential qualities. But perfectionism is something different. It's striving for a level so unrealistically high that you're either so intimidated you can't even begin or you're reluctant ever to pronounce something 'finished'. However commendable the attitude, it has no practical use. You just end up making yourself unhappy along with everybody else you're involved with.

You may believe, as so many do, that perfection does exist. But I'm going to prove to you that in terms of the things human beings do, it doesn't. Oh, OK, if I ask you two plus two and you answer four then, yes, that's the perfect answer. But let's look at things that are a little more complicated.

The test is this. If something is perfect it's incapable of improvement. So let's take a look around. Let's take your TV. Is the picture quality so good it could never be improved? Obviously not. Could your car be more durable, quieter, more fuel efficient? Obviously it could. Have you ever seen a film in which every line of dialogue was convincing, every gesture accurate, every camera angle satisfying and the plot always clear? No. I won't go on. When you think about it you'll see that perfection of that kind doesn't exist.

Possibly you fear that if you don't deliver perfection you'll get the sack. I've got news for you. If you think you've been delivering perfection up till now you're mistaken. But, of course, you didn't really think that, did you! No human being ever delivers perfection. But by striving for perfection and thinking you must achieve perfection you're creating a barrier. In my profession we call it 'writers' block'. It's when you're so anxious to create a masterpiece that you can't actually function at all. Believe me, the people who pay you are going to be far happier if you produce three pieces of competent work rather than one piece of 'perfect' work.

Try it now

Whatever you have to do today, set out to do it to a good and competent standard but not to perfection. At the end of the day work out how much you got through compared with a perfectionist day.

Try coming at the situation from a completely different tack. Try to see that things you've been dismissing as imperfect are, in fact, fine in their way. For example, take a look at yourself in the mirror. Too short at 5' 2"? Who says? In fact, you're a fine example of a person of 5' 2". Too many freckles? Who says? In fact, you're a fine example of freckles. Bald? You're a fine example of baldness.

▶ Exaggeration

Have you ever said, 'Why is this always happening to me?' You know the kind of thing. You get a bird-dropping on your clothes and you say it. You get a puncture and you say it. You get a parking ticket and you say it. And yet it's never true. You get a parking ticket once a year, a bird dropping on your clothes once in five years and a puncture once a decade. It's an exaggeration.

So, do you exaggerate the unfortunate things that happen in your life? It would be far better for your IBS if you did the opposite.

As we saw above, the exaggeration of pain in the part of the brain known as the anterior cingulate cortex is a feature of IBS. A link with the exaggeration of emotional pain is not impossible.

Try it now

Instead of focusing on the negative in an exaggerated way, try focusing on the positive.

Let's start with you. What are your good points? I want you to write them down. You don't have to be 'world class' in any of them to add them to your list. Here are some suggestions to get you going:

▶ I don't deliberately harm anybody else.
▶ I always make time for my friends when they have problems.
▶ I'm quite good at telling jokes and making people laugh.
▶ I don't make a fuss when things go wrong.
▶ I'm good at drawing.
▶ Dogs like me.

Now you make your own list.

If you really can't think of anything then you're being too hard on yourself. In fact, if your sheet of paper is blank or with only a couple of points written down then we don't have to look very far for one of the sources of your unhappiness. You don't like yourself enough. You don't love yourself enough. Well, you should. For a start, you're certainly modest. So put that down. You're obviously sensitive. So put that down. You're also introspective. Add that to the list. That's three useful qualities already.

Many unhappy people simply demand too much of themselves and those around them, too. We're all human beings – animals, in fact – with enormous limitations. You're going to have to learn to accept that about yourself and your fellow man and woman. Just do your best. Nobody can ask more. Now get back to the list and don't stop until you've got at least 20 things written down.

When you've finished writing about yourself, make a list of all the good points about your partner. Again, here are some suggestions to get you going:

▶ He/she seldom gets angry.
▶ He/she never spends money without discussing it with me first.
▶ He/she is always very considerate towards my parents.

▶ He/she looks after me when I'm ill.
▶ He/she likes many of the same things I do.
▶ He/she makes me laugh.
▶ He/she cooks beautiful meals for me.

And then do the same for your children, your parents and anyone else you're close to.

Next you're going to make a list of all the good things in your life. For example:
▶ I'm in good health.
▶ I have somewhere nice to live.
▶ I never have to go hungry.
▶ I have many friends.

Nobody's list should – could – be short. If yours is then you've got to learn to appreciate things more than you do. You're taking far too much for granted. You've got to learn to stop comparing with the ultimate – the richest person, the biggest house, the strongest athlete, the most beautiful face – and try to get a bit more perspective. Don't forget there are also people who have almost nothing to eat, who don't have any kind of house and who combat severe disabilities.

When you've finished your lists copy them out very clearly onto some card or, if you have a computer, print them. Also make the 'highlights' into a portable version you can keep in your wallet or handbag. Make sure you always have copies close to hand. Here's what you do.
▶ When you get up in the morning read the lists.
▶ When you're having lunch read the lists.
▶ Just before you go to sleep read the lists.
▶ Any time you're having an IBS flare-up read the lists.

Remember this

It probably sounds a rather silly idea to make lists of positive things, but it's been proven to be an extremely powerful technique for achieving happiness. And the happier you are the less stressed you'll be and the less debilitating your irritable bowel symptoms will be. So do try it. And not just for a day. It's going to take your brain some time to rewire itself with this new and more positive way of looking at the world. Try it for at least a month.

PESSIMISM

Your partner is late. You look at your watch and begin to get angry. A little while later your anger starts to become overlaid by concern. 'He's had an accident.' 'She's been abducted.' You're worried and your irritable bowel symptoms start to play up.

After an hour your partner arrives. What happened? It turns out to have been nothing more than a simple misunderstanding over the time. One of you thought you'd agreed on 8 o'clock, the other 9 o'clock.

These kinds of situations happen. The people whispering in the corner, who – you convince yourself – are saying bad things about you. The boss who doesn't greet you in the usual, cheerful way because – you convince yourself – he's about to reprimand you. The medical test, which – you convince yourself – is bound to have found a life-threatening condition.

In the same vein, we all also like to have a go at predicting the future and enjoy saying 'I told you so' when our forecasts turn out to be right. And the predictions are usually negative. But we tend to forget the occasions when we were wrong. If you're someone who always has a negative view of things you may be surprised how many times that happens. Let's find out.

 Try it now

Carry a notebook with you for the next week. Every time a negative prediction comes into your mind, write it down. Things like:
- I'm never going to be able to do this.
- He's going to cause trouble for me.
- She isn't going to like me.
- They look very suspicious.
- There's no way out of this.
- It can only mean something terrible has happened.

When the outcome of the situation is known, write it in your notebook. At the end of the week tot up how many times your negative predictions turned out to be right and how many wrong. You'll almost certainly find the latter outweigh the former by a considerable margin. That's an awful lot of anxiety over nothing. Now try writing down positive predictions and see how many times they come true. Yes, more often than you think!

Once you've done the exercise you'll know your negative outlook just isn't in accordance with reality. You're wasting a lot of energy, making yourself unhappy quite needlessly and intensifying your irritable bowel symptoms. Look at it this way. What have you got to lose by adopting a positive stance? 'The people in the corner are discussing their sex lives.' 'The boss is preoccupied.' 'The results of my medical test will be fine.' Of course, there are occasions when it would be prudent to take some action, but you can still do that without having to visualize worst-case scenarios. Believe the best until you have reason to know otherwise.

SELF-BLAME

Accepting responsibility for things that aren't your responsibility is a common error, particularly among women. Women are the nurturing sex so it's understandable that they react this way more often than men do.

Let's say that your elderly father insists on driving. He hasn't had an accident yet but you're convinced it's only a matter of time – and not very much time. You feel it's your responsibility to tell him to sell the car. You lie awake at night worrying about how to persuade him – and how he'll manage without it. You're unhappy.

But let's look at the facts. Your father is an adult, with more experience than you have, and makes his own decisions. He hasn't had an accident, which probably means he's acknowledged his limitations and drives accordingly. The police haven't interfered. His doctor hasn't interfered. So why should you?

Try it now

Make a checklist of 25 things involving other people that you consider yourself to be responsible for (for example, ironing your partner's shirts, checking that your partner is 'correctly' dressed, doing the kids' homework for them). Then go through the list asking yourself:
▶ Am I really responsible for this?
▶ Why can't the other person do this for him/herself?

- In what way am I so superior that only I can do this?
- In what way is the other person so inferior as to be incapable of doing this?

Of course, when you love someone there's a natural desire to intervene – and, sometimes, that's right. But you can easily go too far. You're going to have to accept that there are things beyond your control and that other people have free will and ideas of their own. Quite possibly you like the feeling that other people can't do without you and that you're indispensable. That's not a terrible thing. The problem comes when you start to worry, make yourself unhappy over something that really isn't your responsibility, and magnify your irritable bowel symptoms.

'SHOULD'

We all have a little voice within telling us what we 'should' do. (And quite often it's reinforced by someone else's voice, too.) I should cut the grass, even though it's only an inch long. I should clean the house, even though I did it last week. I should go to Bill and Sheila's party, even though we have nothing in common. And when you don't do what you should you feel guilt. Guilt is a very unpleasant emotion to have to deal with. Yes, sometimes there just are things you've 'got' to do, whether you like it or not. But far fewer than you think. Focus on happiness not 'should'.

Try it now

For the next week banish all 'shoulds' and see what happens. Each time you're faced with a 'should situation' apply a different mindset to it: Taking all things into account, will I be happier if I do this or if I don't?

APPLYING THE PRINCIPLES TO YOUR PAST

You can usefully apply the principles of CT not only to the present but also to your past.

But surely, you say, we can't change our past lives? Surely we can't change the facts of history? Well, no, we can't change the facts but are you sure they are the facts? We only remember a tiny fraction of past events and, to some extent, we choose our memories to fit with the world view we've selected for ourselves. Some people choose to remember the best and some choose to remember the worst.

Are you, for example, one of the many people who has been through a separation or divorce? What, then, are your memories of your ex-partner? Can you remember that you once loved him or her? Or can you only recall the rows and the flying saucepans? Do you only want to remember the rows and the flying saucepans? That's most likely the case. But there was a time when you were in love. There was a time when you were happy together. Why not remember those times?

It doesn't mean pretending the bad things never happened. You may, indeed, have to face up to those bad things and deal with them. But it may be that you have feelings of bitterness and resentment that are spoiling your present life and yet which aren't justified. There is a different way of looking back at things. Consider these statements, for example:

▶ I should never have married, but then, inevitably we make mistakes when we're young.

▶ We had some good years together.

▶ We had some difficult times but I learned from them.

▶ It's fortunate we split up because I'm now able to fulfil myself in a more suitable relationship.

▶ I've made my new relationship much stronger than it ever would have been if I hadn't got those past experiences to draw on.

These are all positive ways of looking at the past. You'll be much happier if you adopt the same mindset.

Remember this

Your past can be a rich source of pleasure if you allow it to be. Don't cut yourself off from it simply because a few things turned out badly. Yes, looking back can make you feel bitter. But it can also make you extremely happy. It's your *choice*.

Try it now

Every day find a quiet time to mull over your past. When you go to bed can be a good moment. Re-examine those events you think of as negative and which bother you. Ask yourself these questions:

▶ Were they really as uniformly black as I've painted them? Wasn't there maybe a little grey, too, or even white?
▶ Am I applying standards that would have required perfection on the part of myself or others?
▶ Am I exaggerating the negative?
▶ Am I being pessimistic?
▶ Am I wrongly taking the blame for things?
▶ Is it really the case that I, or others, should have behaved differently?

Try it now

If you're having a problem with a particular bad memory you may be able to desensitize yourself through the power of music. Here's how. Recall the scene and, at the same time, 'play' some music in your mind that is completely incongruous. In most cases you'll want it to be something humorous – perhaps the theme from your favourite comedy programme. In other words, it's as if you're watching a film with the wrong soundtrack. Do this several times. Check your response by recalling the scene again but this time without the music. Hopefully you'll find you're a lot less upset by the memory than you had been.

▶ **Why are we negative?**

It's worth asking why you or anybody else should want to look at things in a negative way. After all, if looking for the positive leads to happiness and if looking for the negative leads to everything bad then only a fool would look for the negative. And yet so many people do.

According to many psychiatrists and psychologists, infants very quickly develop into one of four types, after which it's rather difficult to change:

1 I'm all right and you're all right.

2 I'm all right but you're not all right.

3 I'm not all right but you're all right.

4 I'm not all right and you're not all right.

You can probably grasp right away that the first of these is most likely to lead to happiness and a relaxed view of life. The second will lead to occasional happiness. The third and fourth are recipes for unhappiness, anger, stress – and increased irritable bowel symptoms.

Key idea

Irritable bowel symptoms can lead to low moods and ultimately to depression. CT can be used to combat depression – that's what it was designed for.

Meditation

Meditation is a highly effective way of making you more relaxed. You don't have to follow any particular Oriental philosophy or religion and there's nothing especially mystical about it. Nowadays it's a perfectly 'Western' technique used by millions of people in Europe and America.

Even so, how could it be possible that sitting cross-legged and thinking about nothing very much at all could have even a remote impact on irritable bowel symptoms? Put like that it doesn't sound very likely. Yet the evidence is there. People who meditate regularly say they feel happier, and scientists can measure the increase in 'happy chemicals'. Those same chemicals can calm your digestive tract. Researchers have monitored the brains of people who begin meditating and found that, over a period of months, activity tends to increase in the frontal lobe of the left brain. That's the part associated with higher moods and optimism. Here's a list of the benefits. Meditation will help you to:

▶ restore normal function to your digestive tract

▶ experience inner happiness

▶ refresh and revitalize yourself after your day's work

- forget, for a while, your cares about the past and your worries for the future

- try to understand the nature of the mind

- increase your control over your mind

- cultivate a calmer mind and a more tranquil outlook

- develop a more balanced mental state in respect of a particular issue

- gain a greater understanding of your true nature

- become more totally aware

- lower blood pressure

- strengthen the immune system.

► When should I meditate?

You can meditate at any time. The important thing is that it should be regular and not just when your IBS is especially troublesome. Some teachers recommend first thing in the morning, especially before dawn, as a way of setting you up for the day. Others recommend the late evening, when everything has been done, as a way of unwinding from the day. Still others like to take advantage of the natural tendency to feel sleepy around the end of the working day. But be careful. Sleeping and meditation are different things and although it's easier to get into a meditative state when your body and mind have slowed down of their own accord there's always the danger of snoozing rather than meditating.

Key idea

Find out what works best for you and then try to stick to it. Your body and mind will adapt accordingly and you'll find it increasingly easy to get into a meditative state at the same time every day.

► Where should I meditate?

You can meditate anywhere. But most people like to have a special place and some also like to have particular 'props' to help them get into the meditative state.

As a beginner you're probably best to have a quiet place where you won't be disturbed. Make it a nice place so that you look forward to going to it and come to associate it with meditation. Except for open-eyed styles of meditation, it will help if the room is dim or even dark. You could wear an eye mask.

▶ What position is good for meditation?

The pose traditionally associated with meditation is the lotus position. That's to say, sitting on the floor with the right foot on the left thigh and the left foot on the right thigh, so that the left ankle crosses over on top of the right ankle. The idea behind it is that it's extremely stable so that, in deep meditation, you won't topple over; at the same time, it's not a position in which it's easy to fall asleep.

Fortunately, the lotus position is not essential, which is just as well because very few people can manage it at all, let alone for a whole session of meditation. When you meditate you need to be comfortable. That's vital. You don't want to be distracted by thinking how painful your ankles or knees are.

If you can easily do the half-lotus (only one foot resting on the opposite thigh, the other foot going under the opposite thigh) this is all well and good. If not, just sit cross-legged. In whichever of these poses you sit it's important you keep your spine straight.

Rest your hands on your knees. One way is with the palms up and the thumb and forefinger of each hand touching to form an 'O'. But there are other ways as we'll see below.

Tips

▶ Warm up by sitting on the floor with the soles of your feet together and close to your groin. Clasp your feet with your hands and move your knees up and down like a bird's wings.
▶ Place a cushion under the rear of your buttocks to tip you forwards slightly and thus bring your knees down to the floor.

There are two alternatives to sitting on the floor. The lotus-type position comes down to us from an era when furniture hadn't been invented but, in fact, you can meditate perfectly well sitting on a dining chair or even an office swivel chair. The key element is to sit away from the back of the chair, keeping a straight spine. Just place your hands, palms down, lightly on your knees.

The other alternative is to lie down. Many teachers frown on this as not being 'proper' and because of the danger of falling asleep. But, in fact, it's an excellent position for meditating because it automatically reduces beta waves. As with the other positions, the spine should be straight, so lie on your back with your arms by your sides, palms up, and your feet shoulder width apart. To overcome the danger of falling asleep try lying on the floor rather than the bed so you don't get too comfortable.

Key idea

Don't worry too much about the pose. In the last analysis, the important thing is the meditation not the position. Whatever works for you is fine.

▶ How long should I meditate for?

You could meditate all day. But, in the context of a busy modern life 20–30 minutes is the sort of thing to aim for. The longer you can devote to it the more likely you are to reach a deep state. Nevertheless, even a minute's meditation is better than nothing. And sometimes it's possible to experience a meditative state while doing other things, such as walking or running.

However long the session, the benefits ripple out far beyond it. It's just the same as when, for example, something happens to make you angry. The incident might last no more than a few seconds but it could be hours before you feel calm again. So it is with the positive effects of meditation.

Key idea

Some people like to set a timer. This can work well because it removes any anxiety about not meditating for long enough or, on the other hand, taking too long and being late for the next thing you have to do. But others prefer to let whatever happens happen.

▶ How do I meditate for relaxation and irritable bowel relief?

So you're sitting or lying down. Then what? Different people use different techniques and again you need to experiment to find out what works best for you. Some people, for example, stare at a candle flame or an image or a wall, others repeat mantras, still others repeat small almost imperceptible gestures.

Here's a simple way of getting into a meditative state.

Try it now

1 Sitting or lying down with your eyes closed, notice your breathing.

2 Without forcing anything, gradually slow down your breathing.

3 Make your exhalations longer than your inhalations.

4 Empty your mind of any thoughts of past or future.

5 Just concentrate on experiencing the present moment, which is your breath.

6 If any thoughts push their way into your mind just let them drift past; don't pursue them.

7 When your breathing is slow and relaxed, notice your heartbeat.

8 Without forcing anything, gradually try to think it slower.

9 Notice the sound of your blood in your ears.

10 Without forcing anything, gradually try to think it slower.

11 Focus on your digestive tract and identify any areas that feel bloated or painful or where the muscles are in spasm.

12 Without forcing anything, gradually try to think your digestive tract calmer and more coordinated.

13 Now notice the little dots that 'illuminate' the blackness of your closed eyes.

14 Imagine the dots are stars and that you're floating in an immense space inside your own body which is serene and all-knowing.

15 Let your mouth open into a smile.

16 Continue like this as long as you wish.

Remember this

If you can't seem to get into a meditative state at all, try:

► lying on the floor rather than sitting

► touching the tip of your ring finger against the fleshy base of your thumb as you breathe in and moving it away as you breathe out. As you breathe in think 'so' and as you breathe out think 'hum' – it's a classic mantra

► gradually slowing down your breathing, making your exhalation longer than your inhalation

► letting your mouth fall open and your tongue relax completely and drop out.

► Am I meditating?

Beginners often wonder if they're meditating correctly or even at all. What should it feel like? In fact, there is no precise definition but the stages of increasingly deeper and deeper meditation should go something like this:

► **Stage 1.** Your mind is no longer filled with everyday matters and you sense that you're drifting towards sleep; you're on the very fringe of the meditative state.

► **Stage 2.** As you go deeper, images may come at you from nowhere. You don't actually fall asleep but start to feel as if you're floating. You may feel like rocking and swaying; that's fine at this stage but you'll need to stop moving to go deeper.

► **Stage 3.** You become intensely aware of the functioning of your body – breathing, heartbeat, blood flow – but at the same time you no longer know where your body ends and other things begin. Parts of your body may feel very heavy.

► **Stage 4.** You feel 'spaced out' and quite detached but, at the same time, alert.

► **Stage 5.** You feel in touch with the universe and nothing else matters at all.

The deepest meditative states are usually only reached by those who have been practising for a long time – perhaps two or three years. But you may occasionally experience moments of those deeper states even as a beginner.

Remember this

Remember that meditation is not a competition. Every experience of meditation is slightly different. Just experience and enjoy whatever occurs.

Muscle relaxation

Muscle relaxation is a fairly easy technique to learn. Working around your body, all you have to do is tense individual muscles or groups of muscles for a few seconds and then abruptly release them.

Try it now

1 Lie on a bed with your legs a little apart and your arms by your sides, palms up.
2 While breathing in, clench your right hand, contract the muscles of your right arm, lift your arm a little above the bed then, while exhaling, let your arm flop back down to the bed.
3 While breathing in, clench your left hand, contract the muscles of your left arm, lift your arm a little above the bed then, while exhaling, let your arm flop back down to the bed.
4 While breathing in, bend your right foot back so your toes point towards your right knee, contract the muscles of your right leg, raise your leg a little above the bed then, while exhaling, let your leg flop back down to the bed.
5 While breathing in, bend your left foot back so your toes point towards your left knee, contract the muscles of your left leg, raise your leg a little above the bed then, while exhaling, let your leg flop back down to the bed.
6 Exhaling, suck your lower abdomen back towards your spine and, at the same time, clench your buttocks, then let the air rush naturally into your lungs as you release all the tension.
7 Exhaling, suck your navel back towards your spine, then let the air rush naturally into your lungs as you release all the tension.

8 Inhaling, expand your ribs to the maximum, then let the air rush out as you allow your ribs to drop back down.

9 If you feel relaxed lie quietly for a short while; if you're not yet relaxed repeat the procedure.

To make the technique even more effective you can break the body down into smaller areas – feet, calves, knees, thighs, hands, forearms, and so on.

Key idea

As you release the tension in each part of your body, imagine it sinking down into the mattress.

Breath control

Your breathing reflects not only your physical state but also your mental state. When you're relaxed you take long, easy breaths and when you're tense you take short, shallow breaths. When startled you may even hold your breath for a while. And all this happens automatically, usually outside conscious awareness.

Of course, you're aware of your breathing now because I've made you think about it. That's the idea behind breath control. Everything is turned back to front. Instead of your mental state altering your breathing, you consciously take charge of your breathing to alter your mental state.

It's a physiological fact that if you exhale slowly for longer than you inhale then you force your body to relax.

Try it now

1 Sitting comfortably upright in a chair, place one hand across your abdomen just below your navel.

2 Inhale gently through your nose for a count of seven, feeling your hand moving outwards.

3 Hold your breath for a count of two.

4 Exhale gently through your nose for a count of 11, feeling your hand moving inwards.

5 Hold your breath for a count of two.

6 Continue like this for at least two minutes and until you feel relaxed.

Key idea

Of course, your count of 11 may be longer or shorter than mine. If you feel yourself getting out of breath it may be because you're stretching the count too much. The important thing is not the actual amount of time but that your exhalation should be about half as long again as your inhalation. It may also be that your breathing is too violent. Be gentle. The whole idea is relaxation.

IBS and sexual abuse

Women are twice as likely as men to suffer from irritable bowel problems. One possible reason is that there's a link with abuse, especially sexual abuse – and girls/women are more likely than boys/men to suffer it.

In the USA it's estimated that between 15 per cent and 20 per cent of women suffered childhood sexual abuse. If abuse of adult women is added, the percentages would obviously be higher.

According to Jane Leserman, Associate Professor of Psychiatry at the University of North Carolina, 51 per cent of women who attended a gastroenterology clinic had a history of sexual abuse. A study of more than 200 women who attended a gastroenterology clinic found that those who had been abused had, on average, three times more symptoms than non-abused women, spent more days in bed due to illness, had more disability, more lifetime surgery and more psychological distress.

In another study, researchers found that sexual abuse had been suffered by 10 per cent of healthy controls, 21 per cent of the less severely ill IBS patients and 36 per cent of the severely ill IBS patients.

In one survey conducted in Toulouse, France (Delvaux M, Denis P, Allemand H) almost 32 per cent of IBS patients (62 out of 196) reported a history of sexual abuse. That compared with 7.6 per cent among healthy controls. So there seems to be a clear link (and not only with IBS but with other medical problems, too).

A study conducted at a Veteran Affairs Medical Center Women's Clinic in the USA (that is, for women who have served or are serving in the armed forces) found that 33.5 per cent were suffering from IBS. Of 18 different traumas, 17 were found to be associated with IBS, of which the most important was sexual assault.

It's clear that sexual abuse in childhood has devastating health implications later.

Key idea

The fact that you have an irritable bowel does not mean you were abused as a child. Do not go jumping to conclusions. Based on the Toulouse figures, for every irritable bowel sufferer who was abused, two were not. So it's far more likely you were not abused than that you were. However, sexual abuse should definitely be considered as a possibility. If you *know* you were abused you should certainly tell your doctor so it can be taken into account in your treatment. Your doctor may prescribe antidepressants (see Step 3) and psychotherapy.

Remember this

The damage done by sexual abuse can be extremely serious and calls for professional attention. Do not go it alone. However, there are things you can do yourself to reinforce therapy. Use the techniques described above to increase your sense of self-worth and self-confidence.

The fear of IBS

In compiling this book I took evidence from a significant number of irritable bowel sufferers and found that quite often (but not always) the fear about the consequences of an irritable bowel was worse than the reality, especially in the case of IBS-D. For example, there was a woman who would never go on long car journeys. She was terrified she might have an embarrassing accident. But there came a day when she was obliged to make a four-hour journey in a mini-van with people she hardly knew. She had no problem. Another IBS-D sufferer told me how he had been terrified about making a long flight in a light aircraft (in which there was no toilet) and yet when he did it he had no difficulty.

So it's a very good idea to keep an 'IBS Diary', not just to link symptoms to foods and emotions (as suggested in Step 2), but to get a more objective view of exactly how frequent your more difficult irritable bowel symptoms really are. When you look back at your diary you may find, for example, that although you think you need to defecate six times every day, in reality there are many days you only defecate twice.

Hopefully your diary will give you confidence. Don't focus on the bad days. Think about what you did on the good days and how you can build on that. Looking ahead, be prepared for bad days but always work on the assumption it's going to be a great day.

Focus points

1 In the hands of a competent professional, gut-directed hypnotherapy in combination with standard therapies is the most successful treatment for IBS.
2 You can hypnotize yourself, although you may not achieve the same level of success as a professional.
3 NLP can reprogram the system that controls your gut.
4 Stress may cause an irritable bowel and it certainly makes the symptoms worse.
5 Relaxation and 'happy' therapies, including CT and meditation, can reduce stress and therefore the symptoms of an irritable bowel.

Next step

In this chapter we've been looking at approaching irritable bowel problems through the nervous system. The next chapter is completely different. In it we'll be looking at the way exercise can not only reduce the main irritable bowel symptoms but also boost your mood and, if you're suffering from it, lift your depression.

6

Step 6: Take control of your body

In this chapter you will learn:

▶ *How exercise improves irritable bowel symptoms in at least five ways*

▶ *How exercise combats the low moods and depression that can accompany an irritable bowel*

▶ *How being overweight can increase abdominal pain*

▶ *How you can keep motivated to exercise.*

Human beings are designed to move. We all evolved from ancestors who were constantly on the go. Consequently, the human body just doesn't function well in the sedentary age. If you spend most of your time sitting down – sitting on your way to and from work, sitting at a desk at work, sitting in front of the TV in the evenings – then introducing more movement into your life could be highly significant.

In one of the most important studies, conducted at the Sahlgrenska University Hospital in Gothenburg, Sweden, half of a group of 102 IBS patients aged 18 to 65 were put on an exercise programme while the other half continued with their normal lives. Both groups received supportive calls from a physiotherapist but only the exercise group was encouraged to tackle 20 to 30 minutes of moderate to vigorous exercise three to five times a week. At the end of three months the results were astonishing. The symptoms of the non-exercise group had improved by only five points on average but for the exercise group the improvement was an impressive 51 points. Equally significant, 23 per cent of the non-exercisers said their symptoms had got worse but for the exercise group the figure was only 8 per cent.

In another study, IBS sufferers who exercised moderately for 30 minutes a day, five days a week, had fewer problems of constipation compared with a control group. And a study published in the journal *Clinical Gastroenterology and Hepatology* found that the higher a person's Body Mass Index (BMI) the more likely they were to have gastrointestinal pain. So the science is there to support exercise as a treatment for an irritable bowel.

How does exercise work? Here are five ways:

1 Exercise massages the internal organs, helping to promote normal peristalsis in the gut, releases trapped wind, and may improve the ileocecal valve (see Step 4).

2 Exercise causes extra blood to be pumped to the muscles, thus reducing activity in the GI tract and calming it.

3 Exercise combats stress, which exacerbates irritable bowel symptoms (see Step 5).

4 Exercise is a proven way to increase endorphins and other 'happy' chemicals in the blood, reducing pain and improving mood.

5 Exercise can reduce BMI and therefore the likelihood of gastrointestinal pain.

In this Step you're not aiming to be an Olympic athlete. The idea is simply to be active enough and fit enough to reduce your irritable bowel symptoms. The Swedish research quoted above shows that quite modest amounts of exercise are already very helpful. If you get a taste for it and want to go further still then that's even better.

So let's check your current level of 'irritable bowel fitness'.

Diagnostic test

The first five questions are designed to check your attitude to exercise and health – in each group choose the answer that most closely represents you. The final five questions are designed to make an assessment of your 'irritable bowel fitness' right now.

1 Exercise makes me feel:

   a happy and exhilarated.
   b bored.
   c tired.
   d miserable.

2 I exercise:

   a vigorously most days for at least half an hour.
   b vigorously for at least 20 minutes three times a week.
   c a bit at weekends.
   d by doing the gardening, the chores and the shopping – that's enough exercise for anyone.

3 A person's life expectation is:

    a improved by regular exercise.
    b not extended by exercise – but it might seem like it.
    c all down to luck.

4 As regards the impact of exercise on irritable bowel symptoms:

    a I believe exercise combats irritable bowel symptoms.
    b maybe exercise does help irritable bowel symptoms, maybe it doesn't.
    c it's rubbish to suggest there's any connection.

5 As regards the depression that can be caused by irritable bowel problems:

    a I believe exercise helps a good deal.
    b I have an open mind about the benefit of exercise.
    c I can't see how exercise could possibly help.

6 My Body Mass Index* is:

    a under 19.
    b 19–23.
    c 24.
    d 25–27.
    e over 27.

*For an explanation of BMI see below.

7 My resting heart rate (my pulse when I wake up in the morning and before I get out of bed) is:

    a under 50.
    b 50–60.
    c 60–70.
    d 70–80.
    e 80–90.
    f over 90.

8 After warming up and with my legs straight I can touch:

    a the floor with the palms of my hands.
    b the floor with the tips of my fingers.

c my ankle bones.

d my calves.

9 In one minute I can do the following number of sit-ups:

a more than 50

b 40–50

c 30–40

d 20–30

e 10–20

(Don't do this if you have a back problem. To do sit-ups, lie on your back on the carpet, knees bent, heels about 45 cm (18 inches) from your buttocks, feet flat on the floor shoulder-width apart and anchored under a heavy piece of furniture. Your hands should be on the sides of your head. When reclining you only need to touch your shoulders to the floor.)

10 I can walk half a mile in:

a under 6 minutes.

b 6–7 minutes.

c 7–8 minutes.

d 8–9 minutes.

e 9–10 minutes.

f over 10 minutes.

(Measure the distance along a flat stretch of road/pavement using your car.)

Your score:

▶ **Questions 1–5:** If you answered mostly 'a' you have a very positive attitude towards exercise and will have no trouble implementing an 'anti-IBS' programme. If you answered mostly 'b' you're clearly open to exercise but you need to be resolute in translating that into action. If you answered mostly 'c' or 'd' you have a very negative attitude to exercise – but what have you got to lose by at least trying it for a month?

▶ **Question 6:** The 'magic number' for BMI is 24. If you're 24 or under you're considered to be at a healthy weight (unless you're below 19, which could pose a different kind of health risk), but above 24 is considered overweight. The higher your BMI above 24, the greater the association with gastrointestinal pain. To calculate your BMI, see the box below.

▶ **Questions 7–10:** Calculate your individual scores according to the following tables and then add the four numbers together to obtain your 'irritable bowel fitness' score.

▶ **Question 7:**

	Men	Women
a	23	25
b	18	20
c	13	15
d	8	10
e	3	5
f	0	0

▶ **Question 8:**

	Men			Women		
	Under 30	30–50	Over 50	Under 30	30–50	Over 50
a	15	20	25	13	18	23
b	10	15	20	8	13	18
c	8	13	18	6	11	16
d	5	10	15	3	8	13

▶ **Question 9:**

	Men			Women		
	Under 30	30–50	Over 50	Under 30	30–50	Over 50
a	20	25	–	25	–	–
b	15	20	25	20	25	–
c	10	15	20	15	20	25
d	5	10	15	10	15	20
e	2	5	10	5	10	15

	Men			Women		
	Under 30	30–50	Over 50	Under 30	30–50	Over 50
a	20	25	–	25	–	–
b	15	20	25	20	25	–
c	10	15	20	15	20	25
d	5	10	15	10	15	20
e	1	5	10	5	10	15

If you scored 75–100 for questions 7–10 you're already extremely fit so doing more is unlikely to improve your irritable bowel symptoms. If you scored 50–74 you're not in bad shape but if you do a little more you'll gain benefits in terms of your irritable bowel symptoms, your health generally and your happiness. If you scored under 50 then, in one way, you're very lucky because you're going to improve rapidly once start exercising regularly – you'll notice a difference in your irritable bowel symptoms as well as your mood very quickly.

Key idea: calculate your BMI

Step 1. Get hold of a calculator.

Step 2. Work out your height in metres squared (that's to say, your height in metres multiplied by itself).

Step 3. Divide your weight in kilograms by the number you obtained in Step 2.

Example:

You weigh 58 kilos and are 1.6 metres tall. The square of 1.6 (1.6 × 1.6) is 2.56. So your BMI is 58 divided by 2.56 which is 22.6. That's well under 24 and fine.

If you only know your weight in pounds you can convert them to kilograms by dividing by 2.2, and you can convert inches to metres by dividing by 39.37. Alternatively, you can multiply your weight in pounds by 705, and divide the result by your height in inches squared.

Pelvic floor exercises

Let's kick off with some exercises that have a very direct impact on one aspect of an irritable bowel and that's your ability to control the escape of intestinal gas. The exercises won't reduce the amount of gas but they will enable you to release it when it's not embarrassing to do so. If you have severe IBS-D they'll also help to reduce the incidence of soiled underwear.

Let's just see how defecation occurs. Peristaltic movements in the final part of the large intestine (the sigmoid colon) push waste into the rectum. When there's enough waste to cause distension of the rectal wall the rectum shortens, thus increasing the pressure inside it. The internal anal sphincter opens automatically and defecation can only then be prevented by conscious constriction of the external anal sphincter. If it's not strong enough then some leakage could occur.

The most basic exercise is simply to flex your external anal sphincter which, in effect, involves several of the muscles of the pelvic floor, including the muscle you use to hold back urine when you feel the urge to pee. But when you get really good at the exercises you should be able to flex the external anal sphincter and the external urethral sphincter separately.

Try it now

Exercise 1. Contract the pelvic floor muscles 10 times, holding each contraction for two seconds. Repeat several times a day.

Exercise 2. After warming up with the first exercise, slowly squeeze your pelvic floor muscles and hold the maximum contraction for 30 seconds. Repeat five times per session, with five sessions per day.

Exercise 3. Repeat the second exercise but this time increase the amount of contraction in five steps, holding for five seconds at each intermediate stage and for 30 seconds at maximum contraction. This will increase control.

Exercise 4. Try to isolate the external anal sphincter and external urethral sphincter and exercise them separately.

If you're a woman you might also like to buy one of the Kegel-type devices (invented by Dr Arnold Kegel in 1947). They're inserted into the vagina to provide a resistance and were first employed as a means of combating urinary incontinence. However they work on several of the pelvic floor muscles including, as a bonus, the vaginal muscles themselves.

Remember this

In the USA the National Digestive Diseases Information Clearinghouse recommends Kegel exercises as a way of preventing both bladder and bowel incontinence.

Try it now

Here's another useful exercise if you suffer from IBS-C. Go to the bathroom at the same time every day. The most favourable time is about 30 minutes after eating breakfast (which helps to stimulate the gastrocolic reflex). Don't strain. Simply sit (or squat – see Step 2) for a while. Hopefully your body will eventually get into the routine and prepare itself for defecation at the set time.

Weight, exercise and an irritable bowel

So we've established that there's some kind of association between excess weight and increased gastrointestinal pain. It's also the case that excess weight puts increased pressure on the pelvic floor and tends to straighten out the elbow-shape where the last part of the colon joins the rectum, leading to diarrhoea and even incontinence.

▶ To what extent can exercise burn off pounds?

It's a popular misconception that exercise does very little for losing weight. Certainly, exercise alone won't make much difference in a week or even a month. But you have to think of exercise as a lifestyle thing. It's a question of what it does for you over the years.

To lose 225 g (0.5 lb) in a week requires half an hour's vigorous exercise a day. That may sound like a lot of effort for a very small result but over a year it adds up to almost 12 kg (roughly 25 lb), which is tremendous. That could be achieved by, say, walking briskly to the station every day rather than catching a bus.

Of course, you can lose weight by eating less, and that may also be a good idea. Cutting back by 500 calories a day (equivalent to a sugary pudding, a slice of cake or a few biscuits) could easily result in a weekly weight loss of around 450 g (1 lb). However, exercise has numerous other benefits both in terms of irritable bowel problems and health generally. So it should always be part of a weight reduction programme.

The weight loss potential for various types of exercise is given below. How many calories you actually burn depends on your weight, your level of fitness and the intensity with which you pursue the exercise. The figures given are intended only as a rough guide.

Remember this

Never try to lose weight too rapidly. Apart from anything else, you'll probably suffer low blood sugar a lot of the time which will make you feel miserable. Just focus on a healthy amount of exercise, together with a healthy way of eating for life, and you will gradually come down to and maintain your ideal weight.

Depression, exercise and an irritable bowel

It's only natural that you should feel, at the very least, fed up with irritable bowel problems. You may even be depressed.

That's where exercise has another role to play. Exercise is fun. Yes, fun – F. U. N. There's no surer way to boost your mood both immediately and in the longer term.

Scientists can measure these things. And they've found that the levels of what might be called 'happy chemicals' shoot up when you exercise.

What's more, exercise isn't only exhilarating at the time. Regular exercise has an enduring effect that also helps keep you smiling through life's little crises (including bowel flare-ups).

Exercise is so good at improving mood that, in the UK, the National Institute for Health and Clinical Excellence (NICE) recommends exercise and psychotherapy rather than antidepressants as the first line of treatment for mild depression. In fact, it's beneficial for all types of depression. In carefully controlled trials, exercise has performed just as well as antidepressants in combating depression, but without the side-effects of drugs.

So why should exercise feel so good? When you think about it, it's not hard to understand how human beings evolved that way. Our ancestors had to be capable of vigorous activity if they were to eat. When their muscles screamed for respite, those whose bodies produced chemicals to ease the pain were the ones who ran down the prey and got the food. Logically, they were also the ones evolution selected. Well, that's a simplistic way of putting it but right in essence. Nowadays we only have to be capable of lifting a can off a shelf but our bodies remain unchanged. So if we want to enjoy those same chemicals we have to exercise. Here are some of the chemicals that reduce pain and improve mood:

▶ **Endorphins.** The word means 'endogenous morphine', that's to say, morphine-like substances produced by the body. Endorphins combat pain, promote happiness and are one of the ingredients in the 'runner's high'.

▶ **Phenylethylamine (PEA).** This chemical is also found in chocolate as well as some fizzy drinks. Researchers at Rush University and the Center for Creative Development, Chicago, have demonstrated that PEA is a powerful antidepressant. Meanwhile, scientists at Nottingham Trent

University in the UK have shown that PEA levels increase significantly following exercise.

▶ **Noradrenaline/norepinephrine (NE).** When generated by exercise, noradrenaline tends to make you feel happy, confident, positive and expansive.

▶ **Serotonin.** The link with exercise isn't so strong for this one but serotonin is a neurotransmitter for happiness and there's reason to think exercise elevates its level in the brain.

In addition, exercise lowers the level of:

▶ **Cortisol.** A stress hormone, cortisol is linked with low mood.

There are also two further processes at work:

▶ **Thermogenics.** Exercise increases the body's core temperature, which in turn relaxes muscles, including those along the GI tract, which in turn induces a feeling of tranquillity.

▶ **Right brain/Left brain.** Repetitive physical activities such as jogging 'shut down' the left side of the brain (logical thought), freeing up the right brain (creative thought). It's a kind of meditation and it's why solutions to seemingly intractable problems often appear 'by magic' when exercising. Being in right brain mode more often tends to reduce stress.

The exercise bonus

But it doesn't stop there. People who exercise a little every week enjoy two extra years of life compared with the couch potatoes. And people who exercise a little more – but still only moderately – enjoy almost four extra years. Those who exercise regularly and vigorously gain as much as ten years, according to a study conducted by E.C. Hammond in 1964.

In Britain, about four-fifths of people don't get enough exercise. That's an awful lot of less-than-optimum health. Join the one-fifth who do! You'll not only reduce your irritable bowel symptoms, you'll also:

▶ feel happier

▶ sleep better

- have more energy
- look better
- enjoy greater self-esteem
- think more clearly (especially if you're older)
- handle stress more easily
- have a reduced risk of heart attack
- increase your levels of HDL or 'good' cholesterol
- lower your blood pressure
- increase your bone density
- boost your immune system
- enhance your sexual responsiveness
- increase your life expectancy.

Warning

If you haven't been exercising regularly and have any of the following characteristics you should check with your doctor before beginning an exercise programme:
- Over 35 and a smoker
- Over 40 and inactive
- Diabetic
- At risk of heart disease
- High blood pressure
- High cholesterol
- Experience chest pains while exercising
- Difficulty breathing during mild exertion.

How vigorous is vigorous?

The word 'vigorous' may sound daunting, especially if you don't take any exercise at all at the moment. But, in reality, it doesn't take very long to achieve, even starting at zero.

You've probably got a pretty good idea already of what 'vigorous' feels like but let's pin it down a little more scientifically.

▶ Step 1: calculate your maximum heart rate

Your maximum heart rate (MHR) is the level at which your heart just can't beat any faster. It can be worked out in a fitness laboratory but there is an easier and less exhausting (although less precise) way. To calculate your MHR use the following formula: 220 minus your age. For example, if you're 40 years old your MHR will be:

$$220 - 40 = 180.$$

▶ Step 2: calculate your training heart rate

Experts argue about the percentage of MHR that provides the best training heart rate (THR). But most people are agreed that as a minimum, THR should be at least 60 per cent of MHR. Beyond 70 per cent of MHR, exercise would be classed as 'vigorous'. At 70 to 80 per cent you'd be in the zone where aerobic conditioning improves the most. You wouldn't want to go beyond 80 per cent unless you were seriously training to win races. So let's stick with the assumption that you're 40 years old and intending to exercise at the 70 per cent level. The calculation would look like this:

$$(220 - 40) = 180 \times 70 \% = 126.$$

At that level you should be able to carry on a conversation – with a little bit of puffing.

▶ Step 3: discover your resting heart rate

Your resting heart rate (RHR) is the level when you wake up in the morning and before you get out of bed. It's the measure of how well your exercise programme is going. The average RHR for men is 60 to 80 beats per minute while for women it's somewhat higher at 70 to 90 beats a minute.

If you're at 100 beats or more you're clearly not getting sufficient exercise. You should be aiming to get under 60. Athletes tend to be in the range 40 to 50. RHRs under 30 have been known.

It's not possible to say that your RHR is directly linked to happiness but there is an indirect link. If your RHR starts going down it's a good indication that those happiness chemicals are being produced during exercise. That, in turn, should result in fewer irritable bowel symptoms.

Remember this

Don't feel despondent if you have a fairly high RHR right now. In a way you're lucky because you should be able to reduce your RHR much faster than someone who's fitter. In fact, you should see it go down by one beat per minute per week during the first ten weeks of an exercise programme (such as the one given below). In other words, you'll be able to see quick results and that's very good for motivation.

Try it now

The easiest place to take your pulse is to one side of your Adam's apple. Just press gently with three fingers and you'll feel it. Another place is on your wrist. Turn your hand palm upwards and place four fingers of your other hand lengthwise with your little finger at the base of your thumb. You should feel the pulse either under your forefinger or middle finger. Count for 15 seconds and multiply by four. However, it's not very easy taking your pulse accurately while you're exercising. A better idea is to buy a heart rate monitor with a watch-style display on your wrist. They're available quite cheaply in sports equipment shops.

How long and how often?

For irritable bowel relief you really need to exercise every day. But it doesn't have to be for very long.

When it comes to painkilling chemicals, the good news is that surprisingly little exercise makes a big difference. Let's take a look:

▶ **Endorphins:** the level of beta-endorphins, the chemicals the body releases to combat pain, increases five times after 12 minutes of vigorous exercise.

▶ **Phenylethylamine (PEA):** the researchers at Nottingham Trent University found that running at 70 per cent of maximum heart rate (MHR – see below) for 30 minutes increased the level of phenylacetic acid in the urine (a marker for phenylethylamine) by 77 per cent.

▶ **Noradrenaline/norepinephrine (NE):** this increases up to ten times following eight minutes of vigorous exercise.

So it would seem that around ten minutes of vigorous exercise is already highly beneficial in terms of endorphins and NE but that PEA levels are slower to augment.

More exercise, within reason, will bring additional benefits. Dr James Blumenthal carried out a study on 150 depressed people, aged 50 or over, at Duke University in 1999. Not only did exercise substantially improve mood but Dr Blumenthal concluded that for each 50-minute increment of exercise, there was an accompanying 50 per cent reduction in relapse rate.

Generally irritable bowel sufferers feel okay first thing in the morning. But as lunch follows breakfast, and dinner follows lunch, so food and gas build up in the digestive tract. By late evening the discomfort and pain may be at their worst. So that may be a good time to exercise to encourage normal peristalsis and to release trapped wind. But exercise is beneficial at any time.

What type of exercise?

The best kinds of exercise for an irritable bowel are those that shake you up a bit (such as jogging) to promote peristalsis and release trapped wind, and those that promote tranquillity (such as yoga) to reduce the stress that exacerbates symptoms.

Below are some suggestions but there are plenty of other things you can do – for maximum benefit aim to keep your heart beating at your THR for 20 minutes. It's important to choose something you enjoy and will be happy to do several times a week. It's no good relying on, say, a ski trip once a year or a game of tennis once a month. So when you're choosing, bear in mind practical considerations such as cost, distance from your home and the availability of friends (if it's something you can't do on your own).

Remember this

If you're very resistant to the whole idea of exercise it's all the more important to find an activity that really inspires you. Something that has a point to it might do the trick. For example, rather than run around the same circuit every day you could aim to explore every street within a mile of your home. A different kind of point can come from raising money for charity through sponsored activities.

YOGA

The physical aspect of yoga is all about taking control of your body. From the irritable bowel perspective that's obviously a very good thing. But yoga also works on symptoms by promoting a feeling of calm. You can learn from a book or DVD but it's much better to have a teacher to correct postural errors and to provide encouragement and motivation. There are various 'schools' of yoga. Seek a guru who, in addition to the *asanas* (postures) also teaches breathing, meditation and a healthy diet.

Certain yoga exercises specifically release trapped wind (so you'll probably prefer to do them in private). Here's one you can easily do on your own at home on an empty stomach:

1 Lie on your back on a carpet or exercise mat with your head, shoulders and lower back pressed against the floor.

2 Inhaling, bend your knees, bring them to your chest and wrap your arms around your lower legs to keep them in place.

3 Raise your head and press your chin against your knees so your spine is now curved upwards at the top and bottom.

4 Rock rhythmically backwards and forwards and from side to side.

5 Exhaling, lower your legs to the floor.

6 Repeat until you have released the trapped wind.

As a bonus, it's an exercise that promotes flexibility in the spine and combats stiffness in the back.

Yoga weight loss potential: one hour a day equals 225 grams (0.5 lb) in a week.

SKIPPING

Skipping is a really great exercise for an irritable bowel because those up-and-down movements massage the internal organs, stimulate normal peristalsis and encourage the release of gas. Here are the advantages:

▶ The equipment costs almost nothing.

▶ You don't need anyone else.

▶ You don't need much space.

▶ You can do it indoors when the weather is bad (provided you have enough space to swing the rope).

▶ You can easily set aside a few minutes several times a day.

▶ You can stay close to a toilet.

Skipping weight loss potential: one hour a day equals 450 g (1 lb) in a week.

WALKING AND JOGGING

Walking is a great exercise for an irritable bowel. You can do it anywhere at any time without any special equipment. Make it as vigorous as you can. Swing your arms. Introduce hills (or steps) as soon as you feel able. If you can manage half an hour straight off that would be really good. But the beauty of walking is that you can do it for a few minutes whenever you feel uncomfortable.

Once you can walk a reasonable distance you can start jogging. Jogging is a lot of fun. The steady, rhythmical movement seems to generate more 'happy' chemicals per minute than many other activities. Those chemicals help combat pain as well as the depression that often accompanies irritable bowel problems. Just think about it for a moment. Here are two forms of exercise that:

▶ don't require any special equipment

▶ don't have to cost anything

- don't require any special training

- provide plenty of fresh air and sunshine out-of-doors

- can be done indoors on a machine when the weather is bad

- can be done alone or with friends

- can be done anywhere

- enhance creative thinking and permit 'meditation'

- make progress very easy to measure.

For all those reasons, walking and jogging are two of the very best things you can do to tackle irritable bowel symptoms and low mood. And even if you take up some other activity, walking and jogging are always good things to build into your weekly routine.

Walking and jogging weight loss potential:

- One hour a day walking briskly on the flat equals 225 g (0.5 lb) in a week.

- One hour a day jogging slowly on the flat equals 450 g (1 lb) in a week.

- One hour a day running fast on the flat equals 675 g (1.5 lb) in a week.

Key idea

One of the problems with jogging is running slowly enough. Yes, slowly. Beginners tend to associate the word running with 'going fast'. Wrong. Don't rush. You're aiming for a pace you can sustain over a long period. That means going a lot slower than your sprinting pace. In fact, to begin with you should try to run no quicker than the pace of a brisk walk. If you can hardly speak you're going too fast.

▶ Your ten-week walking and jogging programme

When you were a child you probably ran about all day but as an adult you may not have run anywhere for years. Nevertheless you can still jog for irritable bowel relief – you'll just have to build up slowly. On your first outing walk briskly for a couple of minutes to warm up then endeavour to run very slowly for just one minute. Alternate two minutes of walking with one minute of running until you've been on the move for 20 minutes. Continue like that every day for a week. The next week try alternating two minutes of walking with two minutes of running. The third week aim for three minutes of running with two minutes of walking. Continue building up the running and tapering off the walking until, after ten weeks, you can run for the whole 20 minutes.

Key idea

Let's be frank. Trapped wind needs to be released somehow. It's not very sociable to do so in a confined space with other people around. But there's no need to feel constrained when walking or running out of doors. The exercise promotes the movement of the gas and the great outdoors provides the perfect situation.

Try it now

If you've got a pair of trainers and some suitable clothing why not give jogging a try right now? Walk for two minutes, run slowly for one minute, walk for two minutes, run slowly for one minute...and so on, until 20 minutes have elapsed. Do that every other day for a week and you'll be ready to move to the next level.

GYM

If you join a gym, you'll have access to all kinds of things. The best equipment for irritable bowel problems would be the treadmill, the cross-country skiing machine and the rowing machine. If there are aerobic dance and yoga classes you should consider signing up for them, too. As for the static bicycle, weight-training machines, free weights and swimming pool, they'll all contribute to your general fitness and happiness.

A gym:

▶ doesn't require you to have any special equipment

▶ can be used whatever the weather

- can be visited alone or with friends
- can exercise a wide range of muscles as well as the heart/lung system
- gives access to a professional on hand to advise and motivate you
- makes progress very easy to measure
- keeps you close to a toilet.

Gym weight loss potential: one hour a day exercising briskly on a rowing machine or a ski machine, or taking an aerobic dance class, equals 450 g (1 lb) in a week.

Key idea

In one study of irritable bowel sufferers, the abdomen's anti-gravity muscles, notably the internal obliques, relaxed when they should have contracted and the diaphragm contracted when it should have relaxed. That allowed the abdominal contents to sag down and out, resulting in bloating. In another study of IBS sufferers, one-third could not manage even a single sit-up. So exercising your abdominals in the gym could be a good idea. It has to be said that a study at the University of Sydney in 2001 found no unusual weakness in the abdominal walls of IBS sufferers, nor any abnormal pattern of abdominal wall activity. But strengthening the abdominals is certainly worth a try and will definitely bring other benefits.

Try it now

Why not go *today* to a gym near you and ask to be shown around?

DANCING

If you've hated all the exercise suggestions so far then what about dancing? You surely can't dislike every kind of dancing, can you? Dancing is something you can do alone, with one other person, or with a whole lot of people. You can do it at home in private or you can go clubbing or to a ballroom. You can do it to all kinds of music. So this is exercise you can't easily find an excuse to avoid.

Some styles of dancing incorporate meditation, such as 5Rhythms developed by Gabrielle Roth in the 1960s – a synthesis of indigenous dance, Eastern philosophy and modern psychology. For irritable bowel sufferers that can bring additional benefits.

Dancing weight loss potential:

▸ One hour a day waltzing equals 225 g (0.5 lb) in a week.

▸ One hour a day of jazzercise equals 450 g (1 lb) a week.

Try it now

Put on your favourite dance music and get bopping.

Case study

'I began suffering with IBS when I was in my twenties. I didn't take much exercise and, like a lot of men, felt clumsy and embarrassed when there was dancing at a party. So I began practising dance moves in front of a mirror at home. At first it was just a few self-conscious minutes a day but after a month or so I was polishing my routines for half an hour at a time. That was when I noticed my irritable bowel symptoms had eased. Once I felt ready to unleash my moves on an unsuspecting public my IBS flare-ups diminished from once a week to once a month. I now go clubbing two or three nights a week, and practise at home more than ever. And I'm not overweight any more.'
Herbert (36)

Keeping motivated

Knowing exercise will reduce your irritable bowel symptoms as well as make you happier and improve your health, should be motivation enough. But, unfortunately, life isn't like that. We seldom do the things that are good for us and even if we start out with the best of intentions it's all too easy to backslide. So here are a few tips on keeping motivated:

▶ Try to take your exercise regularly at a certain time or times every day then, when the moment arrives, your body will soon start demanding that you do something active with it.

▶ If your favourite exercise is out of doors try to have an indoor back-up you can turn to in bad weather.

▶ Exercise together with friends and jolly each another along (unless, of course, you prefer to be alone).

▶ Don't strain; take it easy and build up gradually.

▶ Keep an exercise diary and enter your times, distances, heart rates, and so on, together with your irritable bowel symptoms, so you can see what effect the exercise is having.

▶ Give yourself rewards whenever you achieve a particular goal – new clothes, a meal out, a massage or whatever you fancy (and can afford).

▶ Hang up a poster of your ideal body and, while you're tackling your irritable bowel symptoms, why not aim for that at the same time?

▶ Keep thinking of the health benefits – reduced irritable bowel symptoms, lower resting heart rate, blood pressure and weight, fewer health problems generally and two to ten extra years of life.

Key idea

The first few minutes of any exercise are *always* a bit tough for everyone, even professional athletes. It takes time for the body to 'get into gear', especially once you're over 40. And if, as a beginner, you're only exercising for a few minutes then, unfortunately, it's all pain because you never get to the pleasurable part. Do persevere because the benefits will come. It will help enormously if you can find an activity that really inspires you.

Focus points

1 Exercise reduces irritable bowel symptoms by, among other things, massaging internal organs, releasing trapped wind, generating painkilling chemicals and lowering the stress hormone cortisol.

2 Exercise tackles the low moods often associated with chronic bowel problems by generating 'happy' chemicals – the UK's National Institute for Health and Clinical Excellence (NICE) recommends it for the treatment of mild depression.

3 The minimum amount of exercise to get you 'irritable bowel fit' is 20 minutes a day.

4 While exercising you should aim to reach around 70 per cent of your maximum heart rate (MHR).

5 To remain motivated, keep an exercise diary and give yourself rewards for reaching targets.

Next step

Only one more step to go. But it's an important one, and especially so for women. It's tackling the hormones that can exacerbate irritable bowel problems.

7

Step 7: Take control of your hormones

In this chapter you will learn:

► *How hormones affect irritable bowel symptoms*

► *How a simple treatment can resolve one-third of IBS-D cases*

► *What to do if you're pregnant.*

In the West it seems that twice as many women suffer with irritable bowels as men, and that three times as many consult their doctors. From various studies it's also clear that about half to three-quarters of women with irritable bowels have worse symptoms during menstruation, particularly gas, abdominal pain and diarrhoea. One explanation for the prevalence of irritable bowels among women seems to be a simple matter of anatomy, that is, of having two ovaries and a womb that can also be sources of abdominal pain. It seems, too, that women are less tolerant of abdominal distension than men, suggesting that their intestines are more sensitive. But a major part of the problem seems to be hormonal. We know, for example, that following menopause the proportion of women consulting doctors about IBS falls sharply and by age 60 the numbers of men and women seeking treatment for irritable bowel symptoms is about equal.

So the picture that's emerging in irritable bowel problems is one of too many hormones, or too few hormones, but, at any rate, of a hormonal system that's gone wrong. Unfortunately, at the time of writing, there are only a limited number of gut hormone problems for which there are therapies. We're going to start with a hormonal problem that affects both sexes but, first, let's try to find out how much of a role hormones play in your particular irritable bowel symptoms.

Diagnostic test

1 If you have IBS-D, is it:

   a a chronic daily condition but without any other irritable bowel symptoms?
   b always accompanied by bloating and pain?
   c something that alternates with IBS-C?

2 Is your irritable bowel:

   a worse after a meal?
   b better after a meal?
   c about the same after a meal?

3 After a high fat meal do you:

    a have violent and painful contractions of the colon?
    b notice little difference compared with a low-fat meal?
    c feel more satisfied than usual?

4 Are your irritable bowel symptoms:

    a worse when you're nervous or stressed?
    b unaffected by stress?

5 Are your irritable bowel symptoms:

    a worse in the morning and better in the evening?
    b better in the morning and worse in the evening?
    c the same throughout the day?

6 If you're a woman are your symptoms:

    a worse during menstruation?
    b about the same during menstruation?
    c better during menstruation?

7 If you're a woman is your sensitivity to pain generally:

    a higher when menstruating?
    b higher just before ovulation?
    c the same throughout the cycle?

8 If you've been pregnant, were your irritable bowel symptoms:

    a worse during the pregnancy?
    b better during the pregnancy?
    c better for a while, then worse?
    d unchanged?

9 If you're a woman on the pill did you find:

    a your IBS got worse when you started the pill?
    b your IBS improved when you started the pill?
    c your IBS was unchanged by the pill?

10 If you're having, or had, hormone replacement therapy (HRT) were your symptoms:

    a better before HRT?

    b worse before HRT?

    c about the same before and during HRT?

Your score:

▸ **Question 1.** If you answered (a) then you might have bile acid diarrhoea (BAD) caused by a lack of the hormone FGF19 (see below).

▸ **Question 2.** If you answered (a) then you may be producing too much of the hormone motilin.

▸ **Question 3.** If you answered (a) you might have a problem with the hormone cholecystokinin (CCK). The best treatment at the moment is to cut down on fat (see Step 4).

▸ **Questions 4 and 5.** If you answered (a) to one or both questions you may have elevated levels of cortisol. The most effective treatments are those described in Step 5.

▸ **Questions 6 and 7.** If your irritable bowel symptoms are worse during menstruation that's a strong indication that low oestrogen is the trigger.

▸ **Question 8–10.** If your irritable bowel symptoms were changed by pregnancy, the pill or hormone replacement therapy then almost certainly some kind of hormone treatment will help you.

Bile acid diarrhoea (BAD)

If you have chronic diarrhoea that turns out to be caused by a deficiency of the hormone FGF19 then you're in luck. It means you have a condition known as bile acid diarrhoea (BAD) and the diarrhoea can be stopped completely.

According to Professor Julian Walters, professor of gastroenterology at Imperial College London, up to a third of the people in the UK who are told they have IBS specifically have BAD. And BAD can be successfully treated with a daily medicament.

Bile acids are produced from cholesterol in the liver and stored in the gallbladder until they're needed for the processing of fat in the intestine. FGF19 inhibits bile acid synthesis in the liver when levels get too high. In BAD it seems that there's a deficiency of FGF19, allowing an overproduction of bile acids which pour into the large intestine where, through osmosis, they attract water. Sufferers have an urgent need to go to the toilet up to ten times a day and pass watery stools.

BAD can be diagnosed by swallowing a capsule containing something known as Se-homocholic acid taurine (SeHCAT). Scans are then taken seven days apart to see how much SeHCAT has been retained by the body. In a normal person around 15 per cent should still be in the body after seven days. If the scan reveals only between one and five per cent then BAD is confirmed.

The standard treatment is cholestyramine (see Step 3) which makes the bile acids insoluble and therefore unable to attract water through osmosis. The diarrhoea usually ends within a few weeks but it's necessary to continue taking the cholestyramine for life.

Case study

'I began having diarrhoea every morning at the age of 19. Soon I was having several bouts of diarrhoea a day. Over the years I saw several doctors and was simply told I had IBS. Nothing seemed to help. Many years later I was researching my condition online when I came across a scientific paper by Professor Walters. I contacted him and he arranged a SeHCAT test. BAD was confirmed and I was prescribed cholestyramine. It caused sleeping problems initially but that resolved after a few weeks and within three months the diarrhoea was gone.' Judith (64)

Hormones and food

If your irritable bowel symptoms are often worse after a meal, research in Sweden (Sjolund K, Ekman R, Lindgren S, Rehfeld JF) suggests the hormones motilin and cholecystokinin (CCK) are the culprits. Motilin is secreted by endocrine cells in the small intestine and has the nickname 'housekeeper of the gut' because it clears out the gut in readiness for the next meal by increasing peristalsis. CCK is also secreted by cells in the small intestine, especially in response to fatty acids. There are CCK receptors throughout the central nervous system and a further interesting effect of CCK is that it increases anxiety – more evidence of the brain-gut connection discussed in Step 5.

Try it now

As from today and for the next week eat five small meals a day rather than two or three large ones to try to keep your motilin and CCK levels down. For example, eat at 8am, 11am, 2pm, 5pm and 8pm. Your largest meal shouldn't be more than 60 per cent of the size of the largest meal you normally have. Keep the amount of fat as low as possible and don't eat more in a day than you normally would. If you're overweight this would be a good moment to cut back. If your irritable bowel symptoms are reduced continue on the five small meals.

Hormones and stress

Japanese researchers (Fukudo S, Suzuki J) have found another influence on motilin. When faced with difficult situations, IBS sufferers experience an unusual rise in this hormone with a resultant abnormal increase in gut activity. A study published in the American Journal of Gastroenterology in 1996 (Heitkemper *et al*) reported that cortisol, a stress hormone, was unusually high in women with IBS. And an Italian team (Patacchioli *et al*) found that not only was cortisol activity exaggerated but that it was especially high in the morning and lower in the evening. Another team led by Fukudo showed that an additional stress-related chemical, corticotropin-releasing hormone (CRH), which has been shown to cause intestinal muscle activity in laboratory animals, is also higher in IBS sufferers. All of that matches the findings reported in Step 5.

So here we have a hormonal explanation of the way stress may cause or exacerbate irritable bowel symptoms. It's possible that, to some extent, the stress hormones are released in response to the trauma of an irritable bowel, rather than causing it. But the link between stressful situations and higher motilin levels is clear and it can only be sensible to switch to a low-stress lifestyle and practise the relaxation techniques described in Step 5.

Key idea

An irritable bowel can become something of a circular problem. The symptoms make you feel stressed and the resulting stress hormones increase the severity of your condition. As time goes by things get worse and worse. You have to cut into that circle somewhere in a determined way and that might involve a dramatic change such as quitting a stressful job or unsatisfactory relationship.

The pill, period pains and irritable bowels

Many women report their irritable bowel symptoms only began when they started taking the pill. Some women find that one brand causes problems while another brand is fine. Still other women have found their irritable bowel symptoms began when they stopped taking the pill. So there's no single answer for everyone. The only way to find out is to experiment on yourself.

Why contraceptive pills should impact the intestines is not hard to understand. There are basically two kinds, one containing oestrogen and progestin, the other containing progestin only. (Progestins are synthetic hormones which have very similar effects to naturally-occurring progesterone.) These chemicals prevent conception but there are receptor cells for oestrogen and progesterone throughout the digestive system and they're also impacted. Sex hormones can have other effects, too. They affect cognitive functions, emotions, vulnerability to drugs and, crucially, pain sensitivity.

When you're having your period your irritable bowel symptoms are probably at their worst. That's because your sensitivity to pain is greatest when your oestrogen levels are low. Oestrogen is at its highest just before ovulation and lowest at the start of the period.

Taking a pill containing oestrogen can therefore reduce the pain associated with menstruation. Some doctors simply prescribe the pill from the three or four types they always prescribe. But there are now many slightly different options. In the UK alone there are about 30 brands available and each one may have its own impact on an irritable bowel. Another approach is to suppress periods entirely. You can do this via an injectable hormonal contraceptive or simply by taking birth control pills continuously without the usual seven day break.

Ask your doctor to carry out a saliva test for oestrogen, progesterone, testosterone and cortisol. All you have to do is spit into a plastic container during the second half of your cycle. The result will make it easier to select the pill that will suit you best.

Remember this

Contraceptive pills can have side-effects including nausea, headaches, breast soreness, acne, low moods, decreased libido, and more seriously though also more rarely, high blood pressure, blood clots, strokes, heart attacks and gallstones. Risks are higher for women who are overweight, over 35, smokers, diabetic or already having high blood pressure or high cholesterol. As regards the total suppression of periods this is something so new that the long-term effects are unknown.

Key idea

You may be able to moderate the discomfort of menstruation and of an irritable bowel at the same time with a hot water bottle or other warming device on the abdomen (see Step 2).

Try it now

A zinc supplement should not only prevent menstrual cramps but also premenstrual tension (PMT), making periods more bearable for irritable bowel sufferers. In trials, 31 mg a day prevented all symptoms of PMT while 30mg one to three times a day for one to four days prior to periods prevented all cramps. However, the Tolerable Upper Intake Level set by the US Academy of Sciences is 40 mg a day so it would be advisable to remain within that if possible.

▶ What contraceptives can I use if I can't take hormonal kinds?

The pill, taken correctly, has a reliability of almost 100 per cent and other hormonal methods (the mini-pill, the patch, the implant, the injection and the ring) are as good or nearly as good. So if you can't use a hormonal method it's going to be hard to find something else as dependable. On the other hand, the pill often isn't taken correctly. According to one survey, half the unplanned pregnancies in the USA are due to forgetting to take the pill at the correct time or to illness (vomiting/diarrhoea) preventing absorption. So the pill isn't as good in practice as it is in theory, and especially not for under-21s who tend to be more forgetful about it. What's more, in one survey of 1,101 women led by Kristen Jozkowski of the University of Arkansas, hormonal contraception was associated with less arousal, less frequent sex, less lubrication, less pleasure and fewer orgasms. And, of course, hormonal methods have health implications. So looking at other contraceptive methods could be a good thing in various ways:

▶ **Sterilization**. If you're certain you don't want more children this is one of the most effective forms of contraception. However, the possibility of conceiving does increase over time and if pregnancy should occur there's a high chance of it being ectopic (that's to say, the embryo develops in the fallopian tube, which is a medical emergency). Following recovery from the surgery there is no physical impact on pleasure. Female sterilization doesn't alter hormone levels and you'll still have periods.

▶ **Vasectomy**. Assuming you're monogamous it's easier for your partner to have a vasectomy than for you to be sterilized. What's more, the pregnancy rate following vasectomy is one to two cases per thousand women in the first year, which is lower than for female sterilization. (Note that you'll need to use an alternative contraceptive method for approximately two months following the vasectomy until your partner's sperm count is zero.) Your partner will not experience any diminution in pleasure or performance.

▶ **The intra-uterine device (IUD)**. Note that IUD-type devices can be with or without hormones. The non-hormonal version is made of plastic and copper and shaped like a T. It's inserted into your womb (uterus) where it interferes with sperm and prevents egg implantation. Two in every 100 women fitted with a non-hormonal IUD will become pregnant in a year. The downside to the IUD is that it can cause heavier and more painful periods in some women which, added to irritable bowel symptoms, may be intolerable.

▶ **The male condom.** The male condom is a very simple solution to contraception and has no impact on hormones, good or bad. Unlike the other methods described it's also the only one to offer significant protection against HIV, gonorrhoea and chlamydia, as well as partial protection against herpes, syphilis and the human papillomavirus. Two in every 100 women whose partners use the condom as the only method of contraception will become pregnant in a year *provided the condom is used correctly*. However, in the real world, the effective reliability may be much lower.

There are other non-hormonal contraceptive methods but their reliability is significantly less. This is a subject to discuss with a health professional.

Key idea

A reliability of 95 per cent (as with the cap/diaphragm) may sound pretty good but it actually means that out of every 100 women using that form of contraception five will become pregnant *in a year*. Over a 20-year period all of the women (on average) will become pregnant. That's why it's essential to use contraception that's 98 per cent reliable or better.

Try it now

If you're on a hormonal contraceptive and suspect it's causing irritable bowel problems ask your partner to try condoms while continuing with your existing method. If he's reluctant explain that coming off hormones is likely to increase your sex drive. The technique of 'gel charging' may also help. Before putting the condom on he first puts some water-based or silicone-based lubricant into the teat. (Note that oil-based lubricants can damage latex condoms.) During sex the lubricant floods out, creating an intense sensation of wetness. If condoms are a success then you know you have at least one alternative to hormonal contraceptives.

Endometriosis

Between 6 and 10 per cent of women are believed to suffer from endometriosis which causes, among other things, the irritable bowel symptoms of abdominal cramps and constipation as well as rectal pain. The successful treatment of endometriosis may therefore stop irritable bowel problems. Other symptoms of endometriosis may include painful sex (dyspareunia), urinary frequency, a dragging pain in the legs, chronic fatigue and infertility.

In endometriosis, tissue like that of the endometrium (the lining of the womb) grows on various internal organs and has a 'menstrual cycle' in much the same way. Just as the lining of the womb thickens, so this material builds up in places it shouldn't be. And just as the real endometrium breaks down at the end of the cycle, so this 'rogue' material also bleeds. But unlike the womb lining it can't just flush away through the vagina. It's trapped and that's why it can cause such terrible pain. Various organs can be affected but it's when this material is attached to the large intestine or rectum that you may experience irritable bowel symptoms the most. Following the menopause problems cease. Treatments include:

▶ **Contraceptive hormones (see above).** By entirely suppressing the monthly cycle they can prevent menstruation with its accompanying pain. Long-term effects of total suppression are not known but it's thought this approach can be followed for years.

▶ **Laparoscopy.** This is the only way to make a certain diagnosis of endometriosis and is also a viable treatment in mild to moderate cases. It involves inserting a lighted viewing instrument into the abdomen via a small incision or incisions. Any rogue material discovered can be cut away immediately.

Scarring afterwards is insignificant, especially for incisions in the navel. You will be told not to eat or drink in the eight hours prior to the procedure. You may be given a general anaesthetic or the laparoscopy may be performed using a local or spinal anaesthetic. Endometriosis recurs within five years in 20 to 40 per cent of cases.

▶ **Hysterectomy.** Complete removal of the womb is a cure for endometriosis. However, it should only be considered in the most severe cases as it can significantly impact a woman's enjoyment of sex.

▶ **Nonsteroidal anti-inflammatory drugs (NSAIDs).** These reduce the pain and inflammation.

▶ **Danazol.** This is a steroid that can induce a menopause-like state, thus preventing the symptoms. However the side-effects can be significant, including the growth of facial hair and deepening of the voice.

▶ **Gonadotropin-releasing hormone agonists (GnRH-a).** These induce a menopause-like state, reducing or stopping symptoms, but due to side-effects such as osteoporosis, must not be used for longer than six months.

Remember this

Although NSAIDs may help significantly with the pain of endometriosis their long-term use can increase intestinal permeability (leaky gut), causing a new set of irritable bowel symptoms. Ginger may be a better bet (see Step 2).

Case study

'I'd been diagnosed as "possibly" having IBS but none of the treatments I was given had much effect. Things went on for about three years with me having terrible abdominal pains from time to time. Then, by chance, I met a woman who was the same age as me and had the same symptoms and who had been diagnosed as having endometriosis. She was given a laparoscopy and was immediately better. I began a diary of my symptoms

Pregnancy and irritable bowels

Pregnancy is a game of chance – some women find that their IBS symptoms improve, some that they get worse. Sometimes they improve at one stage in the pregnancy, only to get worse again at another stage. You may have terrible irritable bowel symptoms in one pregnancy but none at all in a subsequent pregnancy. After giving birth, IBS may get better or it may get worse. It's all a bit of a lottery. What's fairly certain is that pregnancy somehow diminishes the diversity of gut flora. But which bacteria flourish and which fade away is hard to predict.

The most important fact is that you don't have to worry on your baby's account. There's no evidence at all that women with irritable bowel problems have babies that are abnormal in any way whatsoever. However, if you have such serious diarrhoea that you're malnourished your baby might be also and you should speak to your doctor or midwife about it. Researchers at University College, Cork, Ireland and the University of Manchester, England, examined the records of 100,000 women in England and found a slightly higher risk of miscarriage and ectopic pregnancy (conception in the fallopian tube) among IBS sufferers. So those are things to watch out for. But, in general, irritable bowel symptoms may be a problem for you but they're not a problem for your baby.

Irritable bowel sufferers often don't feel very much like sex, which makes conception rather difficult in the first place. In one study, more than four-fifths of sufferers said IBS affected their sex lives, causing low libido or pain during sex and reducing frequency of sex. However, very, very few women or men report having had an embarrassing bowel problem while actually having sex. It's possible the hormones released during sexual excitement have something to do with it. Apart from which, if you add up the number of hours per day you're actually affected by your irritable bowel problems then, unless your symptoms are really severe, you'll probably find there's plenty of time you're feeling 'normal'. So go for it.

Pregnancy limits your options for dealing with irritable bowel problems. Here are a few tips:

▶ Implement the Seven Step Programme before you try to get pregnant.

▶ The recommended iron supplement (the World Health Organization suggests 60 mg a day) may cause constipation. If you already have IBS-C discuss this with your doctor. If you have IBS-D the iron supplement may help.

▶ In bed switch between lying on your left and right sides fairly frequently to help dislodge trapped gas.

▶ Drink plenty of water.

▶ Ginger is considered safe in pregnancy and will help with morning sickness as well as with irritable bowel problems (see Step 2).

▶ Enteric-coated peppermint oil capsules prevent painful spasms (see Step 2). There is, however, the possibility that in high doses they will relax the uterine muscles along with the GI tract muscles thus increasing the risk of miscarriage. They may also reduce the production of breast milk. If you have IBS-C enteric-coated peppermint oil capsules may make constipation worse but if you have IBS-D they should reduce diarrhoea.

▶ Eat plenty of soluble fibre (see Step 4).

▶ Try gut-directed hypnotherapy or self-hypnosis (see Step 5).

▶ Get plenty of exercise (see Step 6). Yoga is safe during pregnancy provided you stick to suitable *asanas* (poses). Some *asanas* may need to be modified. For example, you can perform a modified shoulderstand against a wall, and a modified plough using a stool to support your feet, and a modified cobra, standing up rather than on the floor.

Remember this

Many herbs, supplements and medicaments freely available for the treatment of IBS have never been tested for their impact on a developing foetus. It's best to play safe and avoid all of them during pregnancy unless they have been specifically proven to be safe. If something worked well for you before your pregnancy and you'd like to continue with it discuss it with your doctor first.

Menopause, hormone replacement therapy (HRT) and irritable bowels

The good news about menopause is that it generally reduces the incidence of irritable bowel symptoms. But what if you try to beat the menopause with hormone replacement therapy (HRT)?

In one study, 40,199 HRT users aged 50 to 69 were matched to a cohort of 50,000 women who had never used HRT. The subjects were followed from the start date until one of the following occurred:

▶ They were diagnosed with IBS.

▶ They reached the age of 70.

▶ They had to be excluded from the study for some reason.

▶ They died.

At the end of the study, 660 women were confirmed to have developed IBS. The rate of IBS among non-HRT users was 1.7 per thousand person years while the rate among HRT users was more than double at 3.8 per thousand person years. This effect was consistent no matter which form of HRT was used, the route of administration or the time it was used. The researchers concluded that oestrogen, the standard hormone in HRT for women, was to blame, acting via the oestrogen receptors in the stomach and small intestine.

The advice is that if you're suffering from an irritable bowel and approaching menopause then you should avoid HRT. But there are other considerations, too, and you should discuss the subject fully with a health professional.

Remember this

Wild yam (*Dioscorea villosa*) is sometimes promoted as a hormonal treatment for IBS as well as problems associated with menopause. However, although wild yam can be used to create the hormone progesterone (a constituent of some contraceptive pills) in a laboratory, *it can't be done in the human body*. There is anecdotal evidence that wild yam works as an antispasmodic to calm irritable bowel symptoms but several scientific studies have found it to be ineffective. Peppermint oil is a much better herbal approach (see Step 2).

Men and sex hormones

As regards men and hormones, an extraordinary study was conducted in Sweden between 2006 and 2007 in which researchers looked at the effects of choir singing (Christina Grape RN, Theorell T, Wikström BM, Ekman R). After a year of weekly sessions, which included relaxation, breathing and vocal exercises plus home study about IBS, both men and women showed a significant reduction in irritable bowel symptoms associated with an increase in saliva testosterone.

Why would testosterone increase? Possibly because the participants felt more self-confident, and also because they were put into a competitive situation. The study doesn't prove that the increased testosterone was responsible for the reduction in irritable bowel symptoms but it might have been. The findings were confirmed by a study conducted at the Southern Medical University of Guangzhou, China, which found that peripheral blood testosterone levels in men with IBS was lower than in control groups.

On the other hand, a study in Iran found that testosterone levels were higher in men with IBS than in a control group. And a study at the University Hospital of South Manchester in the UK found no statistically significant difference between the testosterone levels of men with IBS and men without.

But what the South Manchester study did find was a lower level of luteinizing hormone (LH) in men with IBS. LH is, paradoxically, a hormone that initiates the production of testosterone.

So the role of sex hormones in irritable bowel problems in men is not clear and no hormonal approach can be recommended at this time.

Focus points

1 More women than men suffer from irritable bowel problems because of their different hormones.

2 Chronic diarrhoea in women and men can be caused by a deficiency of the FGF19 hormone which is easily corrected through medication.

3 Hormonal contraceptives and pregnancy may improve irritable bowel symptoms or make them worse (it all depends on your own hormonal make-up).

4 Irritable bowel symptoms may be due to, or exacerbated by, endometriosis which can be successfully treated in most cases.

5 Irritable bowel symptoms tend to improve after menopause but hormone replacement therapy (HRT) makes them worse.

Next step

That's the end of the Seven Step Programme. Your next task is to implement it fully. Be methodical. Don't just pick the treatments here and there that sound easy. Work your way through each step testing everything that's relevant to your case. Keep a diary, as suggested. It will help you identify causes and effects and make clearer what works for you and what doesn't. Good luck!

The author will be very pleased to hear how you fared on the Seven Step Programme. You can contact him via his website www.pauljenner.eu.

Taking it further

Books

First of all I'd like to invite you to take a look at my website www.pauljenner.eu. I'm constantly adding material related to my books and I'd certainly welcome your comments and contributions to any of the ongoing topics. If you've found this book useful you might be interested in some of my others:

Beat Your Depression (2007). London: Hodder Arnold.

From the Teach Yourself series:

How To Be Happier (2010). London: Hodder Education.

Transform Your Life With NLP (2010). London: Hodder Education.

Be More Confident (2010). London: Hodder Education.

Have Great Sex (2010). London: Hodder Education.

Get Intimate With Tantric Sex (2010). London: Hodder Education.

Help Yourself To Live Longer (2010). London: Hodder Education.

From the Bullet Guide series:

Beat Negativity With CBT (Hodder Education, 2011)

Several of these titles are available in abridged form in the Flash series:

Life-Changing Happiness

Amazing Sex the Tantric Way

Kickstart Your Life With NLP

Master the Art of Confidence

OTHER BOOKS

Bandler, R. and Grinder, J. (1979). *Frogs Into Princes*. Boulder, Colorado: Real People Press.

This is the book that popularized Neuro-Linguistic Programming (NLP) and is actually the transcript of a live training session.

Bavister, S. and Vickers, A. (2008). *Teach Yourself NLP*. London: Hodder Education.

A comprehensive and very readable description of everything in NLP by two certified NLP coaches. A good book for anyone going on an NLP course.

Burns, D. D. (1999). *Feeling Good – The New Mood Therapy*. New York: Avon Books.

An excellent introduction to cognitive therapy (CT) and how to use it for self-help.

Campbell-McBride, N. (2010). *Gut and Psychology Syndrome*. Cambridge: Medinform Publishing.

Full details of the Gut and Psychology Syndrome (GAPS)™ diet for IBS as devised by Dr Natasha Campbell-McBride.

Erickson, M. H., and Rossi, E. L. (1979). *Hypnotherapy – An Explanatory Casebook*. Irvington.

This is a much more readable account of Erickson's methods than Bandler and Grinder's *Patterns of the Hypnotic Techniques of Milton H Erickson*. Rossi describes Erickson's techniques in plain language and includes transcripts of Erickson's actual words together with explanatory comments.

Pimentel, M. (2006). *A New IBS Solution*. Los Angeles: Health Point Press.

Dr Mark Pimentel, Director of the Gastrointestinal Motility Program at Cedars-Sinai Medical Center, is a pioneer in the antibiotic treatment of small intestinal bacterial overgrowth (SIBO), one of the causes of IBS.

Shepherd S. and Gibson P. (2013). *The Complete Low FODMAP Diet*. New York: Experiment

Full details of the FODMAP diet for IBS by the leaders of the team that developed it at Monash University, Melbourne, Australia.

Useful websites

http://authentichappiness.org

Website of Dr Martin Seligman, founder of 'Positive Psychology'.

www.gaps.me

Website of Dr Natasha Campbell-McBride who devised the GAPS™ diet for the treatment of psychological problems caused by digestive disorders, including IBS.

http://www.helpforibs.com/

Recipes, supplements, herbal teas, books and advice about IBS as a brain-gut dysfunction.

http://www.ibs-care.org/

Useful information from the South Manchester Functional Bowel Service, one of the world's leading IBS research and treatment centres and a pioneer in gut-directed hypnotherapy.

http://www.ibsgroup.org/

Claimed to be the largest online community for IBS sufferers. Plenty of articles and stories as well as the opportunity to make pen pals and meet up.

http://www.ibshypnosis.com/

Website of Olafur Palsson, Associate Professor of Medicine at the University of North Carolina, a specialist in hypnosis for IBS.

http://www.ibsresearchupdate.org/

IBS Research Update is the website of the IBS Research Appeal, a charitable research programme at the Central Middlesex Hospital in London, England.

http://www.ibstales.com/

Personal experiences and treatment reviews from fellow IBS sufferers.

http://leakygutresearch.com/

Useful information about the causes and treatment of gut permeability.

http://www.nationalcandidacenter.com/

Detailed information about the diagnosis and treatment of candida yeast infection.

http://www.patient.co.uk/health/irritable-bowel-syndrome

Advice from the UK's leading independent health site.

www.positivepsychology.org

Website of the 'Positive Psychology' movement.

http://www.siboinfo.com/index.html

Website of Dr Allison Siebecker, a specialist in small intestinal bacterial overgrowth (SIBO).

www.stressinstitute.com

Tips on how to avoid stress and how to cope with it.

Useful organizations

▶ American Restroom Association

PO Box 65111
Baltimore
MD 21209
800 247 3864

office@americanrestroom.org

http://americanrestroom.org/pr/index.htm

Describes itself as 'America's advocate for the availability of clean, safe, well-designed public restrooms'.

▶ The Bladder and Bowel Foundation

SATRA Innovation Park
Rockingham Road

Kettering
Northants
NN16 9JH
General enquiries: 01536 533255
Helpline: 0845 345 0165

info@bladderandbowelfoundation.org

www.bladderandbowelfoundation.org

▶ Core

3 St Andrews Place
London
NW1 4LB
020 7486 0341

info@corecharity.org.uk

www.corecharity.org.uk

Charity funding research into gut and liver disease, including IBS, and campaigning on behalf of sufferers.

▶ The IBS Network

Unit 1.12 SOAR Works
14 Knutton Road
Sheffield
S5 9NU
0114 272 32 53

info@theibsnetwork.org

www.theibsnetwork.org

The IBS Network is a UK charity for IBS sufferers, providing advice, organizing self-help groups, providing 'Can't Wait' cards and campaigning.

▶ MedicAlert Foundation®

2323 Colorado Avenue
Turlock
CA 95382
1.888.633.4298

http://www.medicalert.org/

Emergency medical support and medical IDs that can act as proof of your condition.

▶ Radar

12 City Forum
250 City Road
London EC1V 8AF
020 7250 3222

enquiries@disabilityrightsuk.org

www.radar.org.uk

Formerly known as the Royal Association for Disability Rights, Radar campaigns on behalf of the disabled in the UK. It publishes a guide to the 9,000 locked public toilets in the UK exclusively for the use of the disabled. As an IBS sufferer you can buy a key through the website.

Index